Bacterial Skin Disease in the Dog
A Guide to Canine Pyoderma

Peter J. Ihrke, VMD

Diplomate, American College of Veterinary Dermatology

Department of Medicine and Epidemiology

School of Veterinary Medicine

University of California

Davis, California, USA

Made possible by an educational grant from Bayer, as part of its ongoing commitment to help educate practicing veterinarians worldwide.

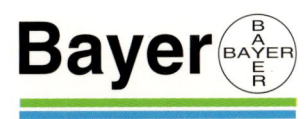

Bayer AG
Business Group Animal Health
51368 Leverkusen
Germany

Bayer Corporation
Agriculture Division
Animal Health
Shawnee Mission, Kansas, USA 66201

Library of Congress No. 95-62464
ISBN 1-884254-30-6

Copyright © 1996, Bayer AG
All rights reserved. Published May 1996
60,000 copies

No part of this publication may be reproduced, stored in a retrieval system, or transmitted in any form or by any electronic or mechanical means, by photocopying or recording, or otherwise without the prior permission of the copyright owner.

The views expressed in this publication represent those of the author and do not necessarily reflect those of Bayer or Bayer subsidiaries.

This manual is primarily intended as an overview of a scientific topic, as dosages are cited for several pharmacologic agents that may not be the same as those stated on their data sheets in a given country.

In addition, dosages are included for pharmacologic products that may not be licensed for veterinary use in a given country.

Veterinary practitioners/surgeons should consult their local data sheet or equivalent for licensing/prescribing conditions in their particular country.

Queries relating to the enclosed information should be addressed to the Bayer Animal Health Business Group in each individual country.

Printed in U.S.A.

Designed and Published by Veterinary Learning Systems

To George H. Muller

Clinical Professor of Dermatology Emeritus
Department of Dermatology
School of Medicine
Stanford University
Stanford, California, USA

About the Author

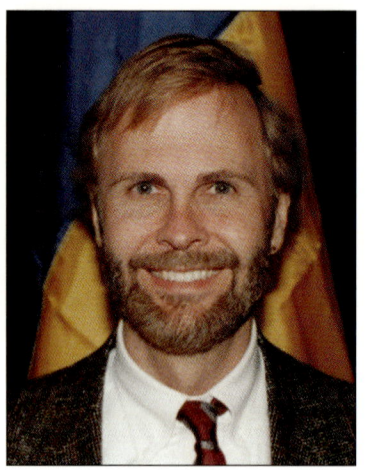

Peter J. Ihrke received his VMD from the University of Pennsylvania in 1972 and also completed a residency in Dermatology there in 1974. He is currently Professor of Dermatology and Acting Chairperson of the Department of Medicine and Epidemiology and the Chief of Service, Dermatology, at the Veterinary Medicine Teaching Hospital, School of Veterinary Medicine, University of California, Davis. He also serves as Clinical Associate Professor of Dermatology at Stanford University. Dr. Ihrke is a Diplomate of the American College of Veterinary Dermatology. He is the author of numerous papers, book chapters, and proceedings and is an extensive lecturer, both nationally and internationally. His current interests include autoimmune and bacterial skin diseases and dermatopharmacology.

Foreword

Pyoderma can cause frustration to both clinicians and pet owners because of its chronic nature, frequent recurrence, and various etiologies. Understanding its causes is a fundamental milestone in the effective treatment and control of this common bacterial skin disease.

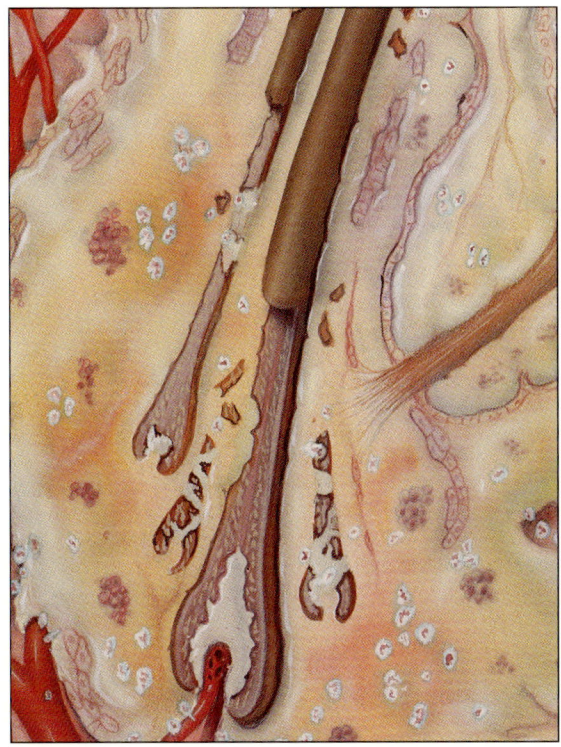

Today's practitioner faces a major challenge in staying current with advances in multiple areas of the veterinary field. Canine pyoderma is no exception. To meet this challenge, Bayer is proud to sponsor *Bacterial Skin Disease in the Dog: A Guide to Canine Pyoderma*, a text authored with state-of-the-art information to update practitioners on the diagnosis and management of this common skin disease.

Bayer has been globally active in medicine for more than 100 years. Our animal health involvement has been ongoing for over 75 years, with research and development leading to the formation of original products that satisfy the needs of veterinary practitioners and surgeons. Bayer's commitment to the veterinary profession, however, goes well beyond the introduction of original pharmaceuticals and biologicals. *Bacterial Skin Disease in the Dog: A Guide to Canine Pyoderma* constitutes one in a series of books sponsored by Bayer that targets areas of clinical relevance in the veterinarian's quest for practical knowledge. This series of publications is an example of our commitment to the veterinary profession through our support of independent researchers in various specialties of veterinary medicine and in the dissemination of information on major areas of scientific interest.

We extend our deepest gratitude to Dr. Peter J. Ihrke, a well-known dermatologist who undertook the task of producing this work, which will surely be an important contribution in the field of veterinary dermatology. A total of 60,000 books will be distributed worldwide, constituting the largest print edition of a scientific book in veterinary medicine to date.

Bernd Kruger
Head of Business Group Animal Health
Bayer AG, Germany

Preface

Enough information, both new and old, is now available to warrant assembling these data in a single resource offering an overview of canine pyoderma. This book incorporates current knowledge of the microbiology, immunology, clinical features, diagnosis, and therapy of canine pyoderma. It is written for busy small animal practitioners seeking to enhance their diagnostic and therapeutic abilities, as well as for residents training in dermatology and dermatologists, who may find the consolidation of this information useful.

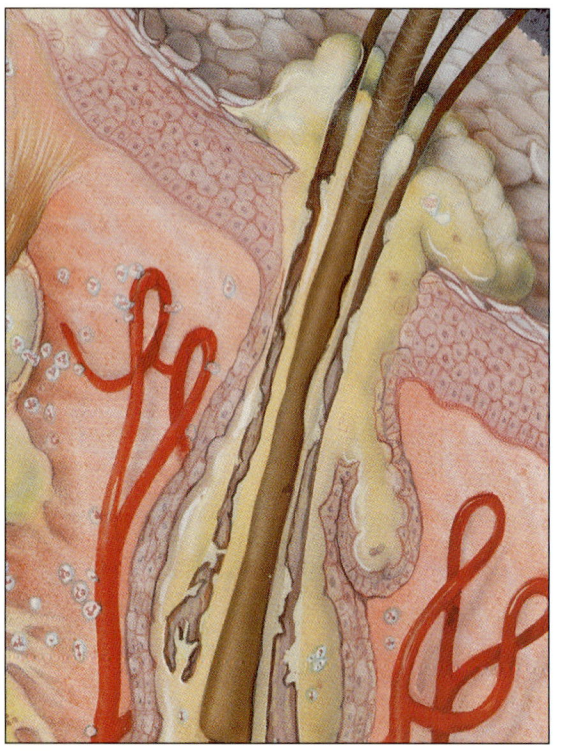

Basic research has led to a better understanding of the ecology of the skin and both beneficial and deleterious aspects of the host's response to infection. At the same time, clinical research has given us new systemic and topical products useful in the management of pyoderma modulated by the perspective of blinded as well as nonblinded clinical trials. This book would not have been possible without the concerted basic and clinical research endeavors of the members of the American College of Veterinary Dermatology, American Academy of Veterinary Dermatology, European Society of Veterinary Dermatology, and European College of Veterinary Dermatology. These organizations continue to foster the investigative attitude necessary for progress.

The author gratefully acknowledges the expertise and organizational skill of Dr. Beth Thompson for shepherding this project to completion, Kevin Stone for superior editorial assistance, May Cheney for the quality of her illustrations, and the Bayer Corporation for their generous support of this project.

Peter J. Ihrke

Davis, California, USA
May 1996

Bacterial Skin Disease in the Dog
A Guide to Canine Pyoderma

Contents

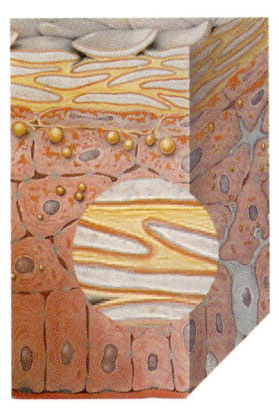

Chapter 1:
Overview of Canine Pyoderma — 1
Frequency of Occurrence/Importance — 1
Predilections — 1

Chapter 2:
Etiology and Pathogenesis — 3
Anatomy of the Skin as It Relates to Bacterial Infection — 3
Normal Microflora of Canine Skin and Hair — 3
Staphylococcus intermedius and Other Canine Cutaneous Pathogens — 6
Alterations in Microflora Seen with Skin Disease — 6
Zoonotic Potential of Canine Skin Pathogens — 7

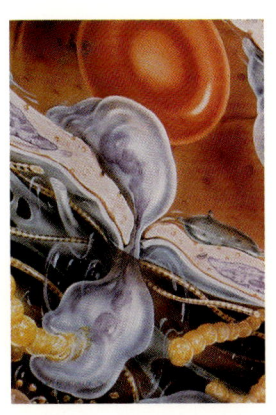

Chapter 3:
Canine Pyoderma—Susceptibility and the Host Response to Infection — 9
Susceptibility to Infection — 9
Host Response to Infection: Beneficial and Deleterious — 10

Chapter 4:
Classification of Canine Pyoderma — 15
Surface Pyoderma — 15
Superficial Pyoderma — 17
Deep Pyoderma — 17
Overview of Diagnostic Differentials — 17

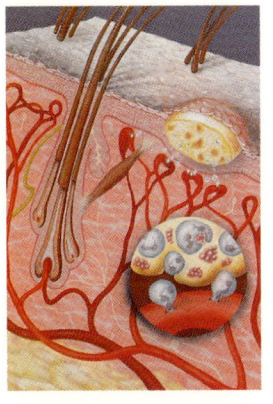

Chapter 5:
General Clinical Findings — 19
Primary Skin Lesions — 19
Secondary Skin Lesions — 19
Overview of Distribution of Lesions — 20

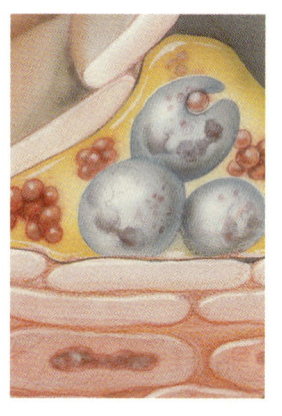
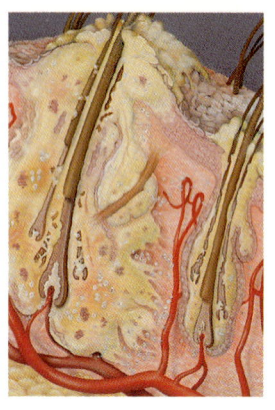
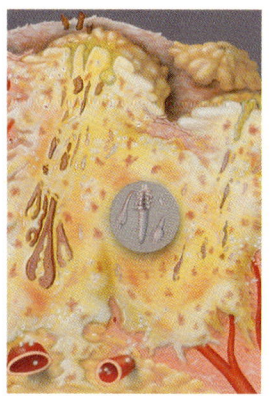
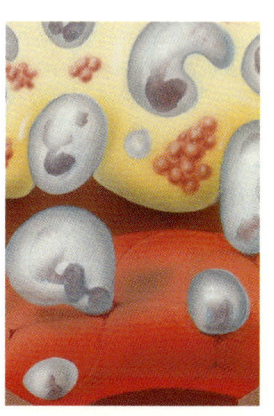

Chapter 6:
Surface Pyoderma — 21
Pyotraumatic Dermatitis — 21
Intertrigo — 22
Mucocutaneous Pyoderma — 25

Chapter 7:
Superficial Pyoderma — 27
Impetigo — 27
Superficial Bacterial Folliculitis — 30
Superficial Spreading Pyoderma — 35

Chapter 8:
Deep Pyoderma — 41
Deep Bacterial Folliculitis and Furunculosis — 41
Muzzle Folliculitis and Furunculosis (Canine Acne) — 46
Pyotraumatic Folliculitis — 47
Pedal Folliculitis and Furunculosis — 49
Callus Pyoderma (Pressure-Point Pyoderma) — 51
German Shepherd Dog Pyoderma — 52
Cellulitis — 53

Chapter 9:
Diagnostic Procedures Useful in Canine Pyoderma — 57
General Considerations — 57
Skin Scrapings — 57
Cytologic Examination — 58
Skin Biopsy — 58
Bacterial Culture, Identification, and Antibiotic Sensitivity — 61
Evaluation for Immunocompetency — 61

Chapter 10:
Overview of the Management of Canine Pyoderma — 63
General Considerations — 63
Systemic Antibiotic Therapy — 63
Topical Antibacterial Therapy — 69
Immunomodulatory Therapy — 71
Appropriate Initial Management — 73
Assessment of Therapy — 73

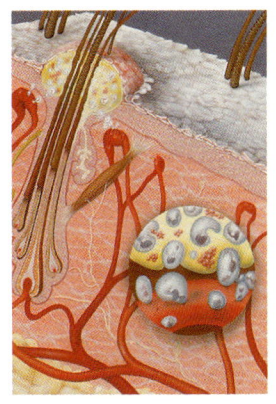
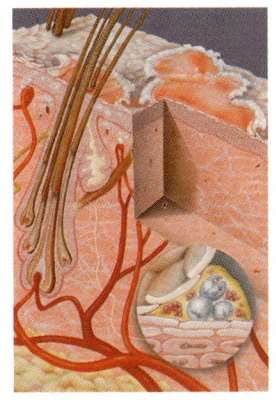
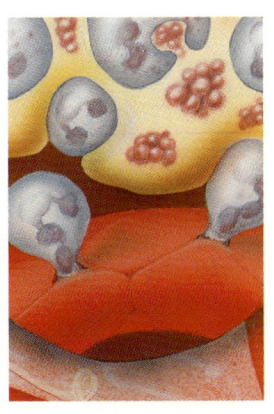

Chapter 11:
Factors Complicating Management of Pyoderma — 75
Inappropriate Initial Therapy — 75
Coexisting Problems — 75
Sequestered Foci of Infection — 75
External Factors — 76

Chapter 12:
Canine Recurrent Pyoderma — 77
General Considerations — 77
General Causes of Recurrent Pyoderma — 77
Recurrent Surface Pyoderma — 80
Recurrent Superficial Pyoderma — 81
Recurrent Deep Pyoderma — 81
Idiopathic Recurrent Pyoderma — 82

Chapter 13:
Management of Recurrent Pyoderma — 83
Management of Underlying Diseases and Other Contributing Factors — 83
Topical Antibacterial Therapy — 84
Immunomodulatory Therapy — 84
Extended Regimens of Antibiotic Therapy — 85

Chapter 14:
Future Developments — 89
General Considerations — 89
Evaluation for Immunocompetency — 89
Manipulation of Microbial Flora — 89
Modification of Host Response — 90
New Antibacterial Products — 90

Index — 93

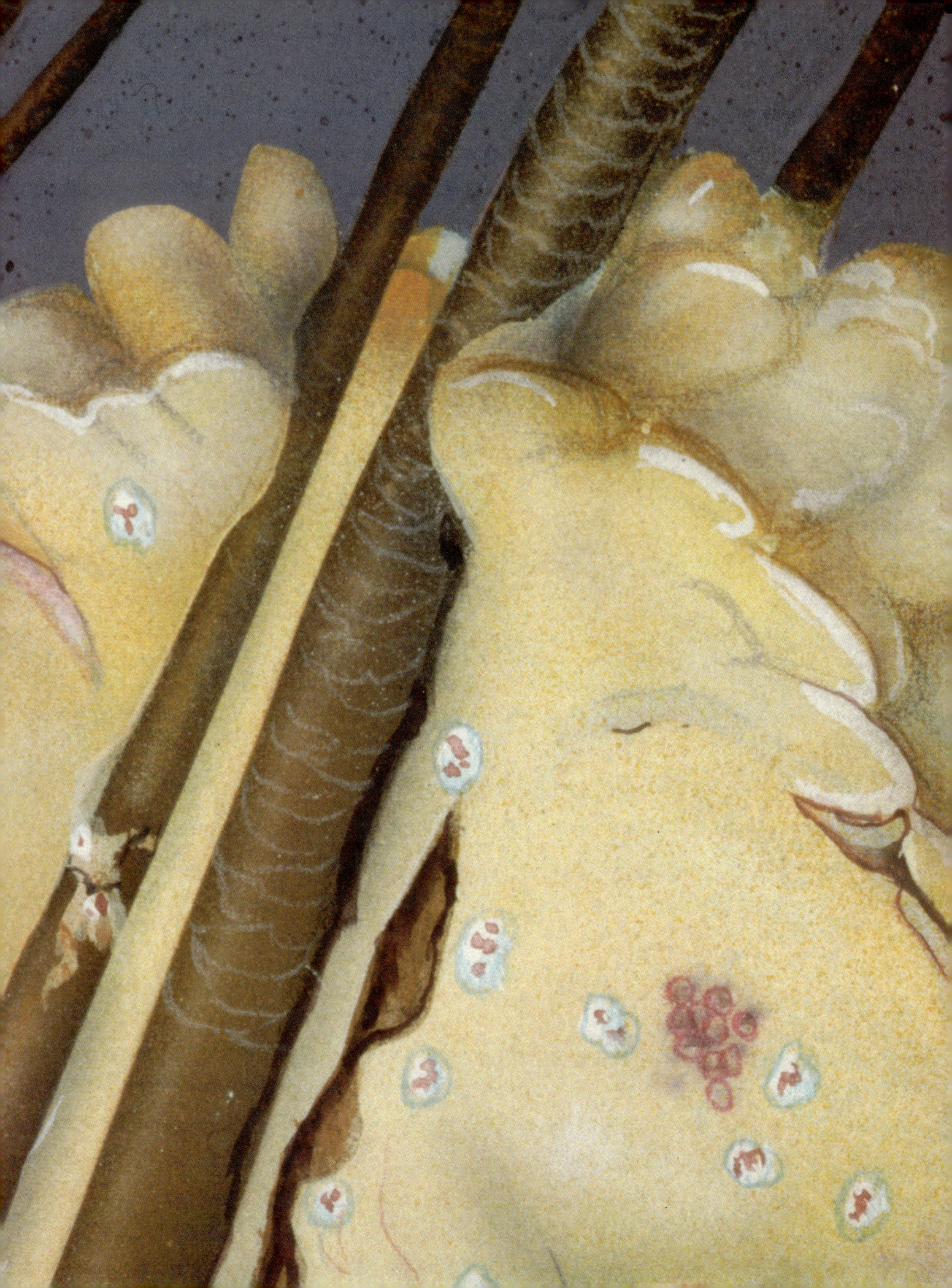

Chapter 1

Overview of Canine Pyoderma

FREQUENCY OF OCCURRENCE/IMPORTANCE

The term *pyoderma* is used to denote a pyogenic (pus-producing) bacterial infection of the skin. Few diseases share the diversity of clinical syndromes seen in dogs with canine pyoderma. The lesions may be quite superficial and involve only the epidermis, or they may compromise deeper structures in the dermis or subcutaneous tissue. Lesions may vary from trivial to life threatening. Perhaps due to this diversity, misdiagnosis and therapeutic mismanagement are common. Misdiagnosis may also be linked to the pleomorphic nature of the disease from dog to dog, in various sites, and at different times in the course of the disease. Frank pus, considered to be a hallmark of bacterial disease, often is not grossly visible; canine pustules rupture rapidly, leading to crusting, and deeper accumulations of pus in the mid-dermis may not drain to the surface. Both the primary and secondary skin lesions seen with canine pyoderma are similar to lesions associated with many unrelated skin diseases. In addition, pyoderma may occur secondary to other underlying diseases or may coexist with other skin diseases. This tremendous clinical diversity makes the proper diagnosis and management of canine pyoderma one of the most consistent challenges in veterinary dermatology.

Little epidemiologic data are available referable to the incidence or relative frequency of occurrence of diseases of various organ systems in domesticated animals. However, it is generally accepted that skin diseases comprise a large portion of the caseload in small animal veterinary practices throughout the world. Published estimates indicate that skin disease accounts for between 20% and 75% of the general caseload in small animal practice![1-4]

Pyoderma is one of the most common causes of canine skin disease worldwide.[5-12] In a large statistical study evaluating data from North American veterinary colleges, the occurrence of pyoderma was second only to flea allergy dermatitis in frequency of diagnosis.[3] In another study performed at the University of Montreal in a relatively flea-free environment (Quebec, Canada), bacterial folliculitis and furunculosis ranked first among canine skin diseases, comprising 25.3% of the dermatology caseload over a 1-year period.[13] Other veterinary sources worldwide either directly discuss the importance of canine bacterial skin diseases on a global basis or indirectly indicate their prominence by space allotted to their discussion.[14-22]

Although it is universally a common cause of skin disease in the dog, pyoderma is comparatively uncommon in humans, cats, horses, and other domesticated animals that have been studied. The reasons for the greatly increased frequency of bacterial skin disease in the dog in comparison to other mammalian species studied are not known. Multiple potential host factors[23-26] that may play a role in enhanced susceptibility to bacterial infection have been proposed, including the comparatively thin, rather compact nature of the canine stratum corneum; the relative paucity of intercellular lipid-rich material in the canine stratum corneum; the lack of a lipid–squamous epithelium plug in the ostia of canine hair follicles; and the relatively high pH of canine skin (Table 1-1). These factors and others not yet determined may contribute to this profound species difference in apparent susceptibility to bacterial skin infection.

PREDILECTIONS

Signalment predilections occur with many skin diseases in domesticated ani-

> The occurrence of pyoderma has been found to be second only to flea allergy dermatitis in frequency of diagnosis.

TABLE 1-1
HOST FACTORS THAT MAY PLAY A ROLE IN ENHANCED SUSCEPTIBILITY TO BACTERIAL INFECTION[23-26]

- The comparatively thin, rather compact nature of the canine stratum corneum
- The relative paucity of intercellular lipid-rich material in the canine stratum corneum
- The lack of a lipid–squamous epithelium plug in the ostia of canine hair follicles
- The relatively high pH of canine skin

mals. Breed, age, and sex predilections, when known or hypothesized for specific subgroups of pyoderma, are given in the sections devoted to each subgroup of canine pyoderma.

Probable breed predilections for various subgroups of canine pyoderma have been published in multiple textbooks, review articles, and proceedings. Much of this information is anecdotal, based on long-term clinical impressions. Intertrigo, commonly classified as a surface pyoderma, is characterized by secondary bacterial overgrowth in tightly apposed folds of skin; because this trait is breed specific, very specific breed predilections are created. In some instances, breed predilections are so profound that names given to subgroups of pyoderma have even included the name of the breed (e.g., German shepherd dog pyoderma).[27,28]

"Strong clinical impressions" of breed predilections are listed in the latest edition of *Muller & Kirk's Small Animal Dermatology*.[29] Of the 70 breeds of dogs listed in breed predilection tables, 26 are indicated as being predisposed to various pyodermas! The breeds listed as most likely to develop various pyodermas include the basset hound, Boston terrier, boxer, bullmastiff, mastiff, Chesapeake Bay retriever, collie, dachshund, dalmatian, Doberman pinscher, English bulldog, German shepherd, golden retriever, Great Dane, Great Pyrenees, Irish setter, Labrador retriever, Newfoundland, Old English sheepdog, Pekingese, Chinese shar-pei, Shetland sheepdog, cocker spaniel, springer spaniel, Saint Bernard, and Scottish terrier. Tables of this type offer breed-based clues to differential diagnosis, which can help in the prioritization of index of suspicion. However, the author has seen examples of pyoderma in virtually every breed of dog presented in veterinary medical teaching hospitals.

REFERENCES

1. Kral F, Novak BJ: *Veterinary Dermatology*. Philadelphia, JB Lippincott, 1953, pp viii–ix.
2. Schwartzman RM, Orkin MA: *A Comparative Study of Skin Disease in Dogs and Man*. Springfield, MA, Charles C Thomas, 1982, pp 5–7.
3. Sisco WM, Ihrke PJ, Franti CE: Regional distribution of the common skin diseases in dogs. *JAVMA* 195:752–756, 1989.
4. Ihrke PJ: Global veterinary dermatology, in Parish LC, Millikan LE, Amer M, et al (eds): *Global Dermatology: Diagnosis and Management According to Geography, Climate, and Culture*. New York, Springer-Verlag, 1995, pp 103–110.
5. Scott DW, Miller WH, Griffin CE: *Muller & Kirk's Small Animal Dermatology*, ed 5. Philadelphia, WB Saunders, 1995, pp ix–x.
6. Ihrke PJ: The management of canine pyodermas, in Kirk RW (ed): *Current Veterinary Therapy VIII*. Philadelphia, WB Saunders, 1983, pp 505–517.
7. White SD, Ihrke PJ: Pyoderma, in Nesbitt GH (ed): *Dermatology—Contemporary Issues in Small Animal Practice*. New York, Churchill Livingstone, 1987, pp 95–121.
8. Ihrke PJ: An overview of bacterial skin disease in the dog. *Br Vet J* 433:112–118, 1987.
9. Ihrke PJ: Bacterial infections of the skin, in Greene CE (ed): *Infectious Diseases of the Dog and Cat*. Philadelphia, WB Saunders, 1990, pp 72–79.
10. Mason IS: Canine pyoderma. *J Small Anim Pract* 32:381–386, 1991.
11. Scott DW, Miller WH, Griffin CE: *Muller & Kirk's Small Animal Dermatology*, ed 5. Philadelphia, WB Saunders, 1995, pp 279–328.
12. Fourrier P, Carlotti D, Magnol J-P, et al: Les pyodermites du chien. *Prat Med Chirurg Anim Compag* 23(6):1–539, 1988.
13. Scott DW, Paradis M: A survey of canine and feline skin disorders seen in a university practice: Small Animal Clinic, University of Montreal, Saint-Hyacinthe, Quebec (1987–1988). *Can Vet J* 31:830–834, 1990.
14. Lloyd DH, Guaguere E: Diagnostic bacteriologique en dermatologie, in Guaguere E (ed): *Techniques diagnostiques en dermatologie des carnivores*, Paris, PMCAC Editions, 1991, pp 91–98.
15. Grant DI: *Skin Diseases in the Dog and Cat*. Oxford, Blackwell Scientific Publications, 1986, p 8.
16. Willemse T: *Clinical Dermatology of Dogs and Cats: A Guide to Diagnosis*. London, Lea & Febiger, 1991, pp 2–16.
17. Mason I: Pustules and crusted papules, in Locke PH, Harvey RG, Mason IS (eds): *Manual of Small Animal Dermatology*. Gloucestershire, BSAVA, 1993, pp 60–64.
18. Wilkinson GT, Harvey RG: *Color Atlas of Small Animal Dermatology: A Guide to Diagnosis*, ed 2. London, Wolfe, 1994, pp 89–107.
19. Fondati A, Ferrer L: *Atlante di Dermatologia dei Piccoli Animali*. Cremona, Edizioni SCIVAC, 1993, pp 14–26.
20. Ohlen B: *Vanliga Hudsjukdomar hos Hund och Katt*. Stockholm, Derma Service, 1988, pp 32–54.
21. Bussieras J, Chermette R, Bourdeau P: *Dermatologie des carnivores domestiques*. L'Ecole D'Alfort, Tome 160, No 5, 1984, pp 428–429, 438, 473–477.
22. Ogata M: *Atlas of Canine and Feline Dermatoses: Diagnosis and Treatment*. Tokyo, Sansuishobo, 1989, pp 7–89.
23. Lloyd DH, Garthwaite G: Epidermal structure and surface topography of canine skin. *Res Vet Sci* 33:99–104, 1982.
24. Mason IS, Lloyd DH: Scanning electron microscopical studies of the living epidermis and stratum corneum of dogs, in Ihrke PJ, Mason IS, White SD (eds): *Advances in Veterinary Dermatology*, vol 2. Oxford, Pergamon, 1993, pp 131–139.
25. Draize JH: The determination of the pH of the skin of man and common laboratory animals. *J Invest Dermatol* 5:77–85, 1942.
26. Roy WE: Role of the sweat glands in eczema of dogs: A preliminary report. *JAVMA* 124:51–54, 1954.
27. Wisselink MA, Willemse A, Koenan JP: Deep pyoderma in the German shepherd dog. *JAAHA* 21:773–777, 1985.
28. Krick SA, Scott DW: Bacterial folliculitis, furunculosis and cellulitis in the German shepherd dog: A retrospective analysis of 17 cases. *JAAHA* 25:23–30, 1989.
29. Scott DW, Miller WH, Griffin CE: *Muller & Kirk's Small Animal Dermatology*, ed 5. Philadelphia, WB Saunders, 1995, pp 61–66.

Chapter 2

Etiology and Pathogenesis

ANATOMY OF THE SKIN AS IT RELATES TO BACTERIAL INFECTION

As discussed in Chapter 1, bacterial skin disease is seen much more frequently in the dog than in any other mammalian species. Most of the known host factors potentially incriminated as contributing to this increased susceptibility to pyoderma are anatomic differences from other species.[1,2]

The thin, compact canine stratum corneum (Figure 2-1)—with its sparse, lipid-rich intercellular material—may present a less efficient epidermal barrier to potential bacterial invasion of the epidermis between hair follicles, leading to an increased frequency of surface bacterial infection (acute moist dermatitis and intertrigo) and non-follicular epidermal infection (impetigo).

Superficial infections of the hair follicle are the most common group of bacterial skin diseases in the dog.[3-7] Consequently, the hair follicle must be considered the most likely cutaneous portal of entry of bacteria in this species. Mason and Lloyd have speculated that a lack of a coherent lipid–squamous epithelium plug in the ostia of canine hair follicles may contribute to the relative frequency of superficial folliculitis in the dog.[2]

NORMAL MICROFLORA OF CANINE SKIN AND HAIR

The microbial flora of the skin is composed of both resident and transient bacteria. Resident bacteria multiply on the skin surface and in hair follicles; maintain a static, consistent population; and are considered to be harmless commensals. Transient bacteria presumably seed the skin from the environment or mucous membranes and under normal circumstances cannot effectively compete with the established resident flora to secure an ecologic niche.

The total number of resident bacteria found on normal canine skin is not large. Ihrke and others found a geometric mean of only 329 organisms/cm^2 in 15 normal dogs (prospective Seeing Eye® dogs).[8] Krogh and Kristensen examined the bacterial flora of 10 dogs (privately owned pets in "good general health" and without skin disease) and found that *Micrococcus,* α-hemolytic streptococci, and *Acinetobacter* were found consistently and uniformly such that they probably belong to the resident flora of canine skin.[9] A later study confirmed these findings, and aerobic diphtheroids were added to the list of probable resident flora. Anaerobic cultures from the skin of normal dogs have indicated the presence of *Clostridium perfringens* in such small numbers that this bacterium probably should not be considered as belonging to the resident flora.[8] Recently, Harvey and others anaerobically cultured a propionibacterium with cultural and biochemical similarities to *Propionibacterium acnes* from 11 normal dogs (euthanatized for reasons other than skin disease) using a medium developed for fastidious organisms.[10]

The coagulase-positive staphylococci isolated by Krogh and Kristensen were the only isolates from normal dog skin considered as pathogens capable of causing canine pyoderma. The initial two surveys were published before the revised classification scheme (categorizing the coagulase-positive staphylococci responsible for most animal diseases formerly termed *Staphylococcus aureus* as *Staphylococcus intermedius*) proposed by Hajek and Marsalek had achieved universal acceptance.[11,12] For clarity, the coagulase-positive staphylococci isolated from canine skin described incorrectly as *Staphylococcus aureus* in older papers will be referred to here with the appropriate name, *Staphylococcus intermedius.*

The participation of coagulase-positive staphylococci in the normal flora of the canine skin and hair coat remains

> Superficial infections of the hair follicle are the most common group of bacterial skin diseases in the dog.

controversial. Hearst reported that *S. intermedius* could be cultured from the nonclipped forehead hair of all 100 normal dogs (from pet shops) sampled in his study.[13] Ihrke and others failed to culture this pathogen from the clipped skin of the rump and dorsal thoracic region of 15 prospective Seeing Eye® dogs free of skin disease.[8] Utilizing the technique initially devised by Hearst, White and others cultured *S. intermedius* from 18 of 20 normal dogs (privately owned pets). They suggested that the populations of organisms on the hair coat might be separate and distinct from the population on the underlying skin and that these organisms might act as a reservoir, potentially seeding the underlying skin.[14] Kwochka used quantitative bacterial assays on 15 normal dogs (living conditions or source of the dogs was not indicated) to evaluate for staphylococcal populations on both skin and hair coat. *S. intermedius* was isolated from 28% of the hair sites and from 20% of the skin sites, usually in small numbers. No significant differences between the staphylococcal populations on the skin and the hair coats were observed.[15] Berg and others isolated coagulase-positive staphylococci from 36 of 44 healthy dogs but, unfortunately, did not indicate whether the hair had been removed from the cultured sites before sampling.[16] Some of the apparent dichotomies could be explained by the varied environments (laboratories, pet shops, private homes) of the different groups of dogs as well as differences in sampling techniques and sites selected.

In an attempt to alleviate the confusion with respect to the presence of *S. intermedius* on the skin and hair of normal dogs, Allaker and others recently evaluated the occurrence of this organism on both the hair and skin of 10 normal dogs (living conditions or source of the dogs was not indicated).[17] *S. intermedius* was isolated from the skin in small numbers (<6 colony-forming units/cm^2) from a minority of the cases sampled. Staphylococci also were isolated from the distal hair coat, and population sizes and frequencies tended to be greater than those of the underlying skin surface.[17] In humans, it has been suggested that populations of bacteria on hair are transients from the environment rather than true residents and that the hair may act as a "trap" for bacteria.[18-20] Dryness and a lack of nutrient supply on the distal hairs also suggest a poor environment for bacterial replication and hence residency status.

Devriese and De Pelsmaecker examined multiple sites of skin and mucous membranes in 50 normal dogs (privately owned pets) and isolated *S. intermedius* from 46 of 50 dogs. Nearly 50% of the dogs carried heavy anal populations; a small group exhibited heavy carriage in the nares. The authors hypothesized that (similar to in humans) the anus and the nares are carrier sites for coagulase-positive staphylococci in the dog and that these regions act as carrier sites for seeding of the hair coat and skin.[21] A subsequent study of 20 dogs by Allaker and others showed similar results.[22] This theory is partially corroborated by an additional study indicating that counts of *S. intermedius* in bitches and their puppies rise in the mouth and on abdominal skin after whelping, which is perhaps associated with increased grooming activity.[23]

As part of a larger study, Lloyd and others quantitatively examined staphylococcal carriage on the ventral abdomen, nasal vestibulum, and the perianal skin of 9 normal dogs.[24] Coagulase-positive staphylococci were found only on one abdominal site on each of 3 of the 9 dogs. However, counts on local sites on 2 dogs were relatively high, leading the authors to speculate that restricted, local colonization rather than simple contamination might be occurring. This indicates that "on normal dog's skin, *S. intermedius* may behave as a nomad, taking advantage of transient changes in the local microenvironment which permit short-term proliferation."[24]

Together, these combined data suggest that *S. intermedius* is probably a contaminant on normal canine hair and either a contaminant or a transient, restricted local colonist on normal canine skin rather than a true resident. In addition, mucous membranes such as the anus and nares are probably sites of potentially pathogenic bacteri-

> Mucous membranes such as the anus and nares are probably sites of potentially pathogenic bacterial carriage.

FIGURE 2-1 *Canine epidermis.* (1) *The thin stratum corneum of canine skin, composed of* (2) *dead keratinocytes and* (3) *sparse intercellular lipids, may account for a less efficient epidermal barrier against bacterial invasion than is seen in other species, leading to an increased frequency of pyoderma. (From White PD:* Essential Fatty Acids in Veterinary Medicine. *Leverkusen, Germany, Bayer AG, 1995, p 19. Modified with permission.)*

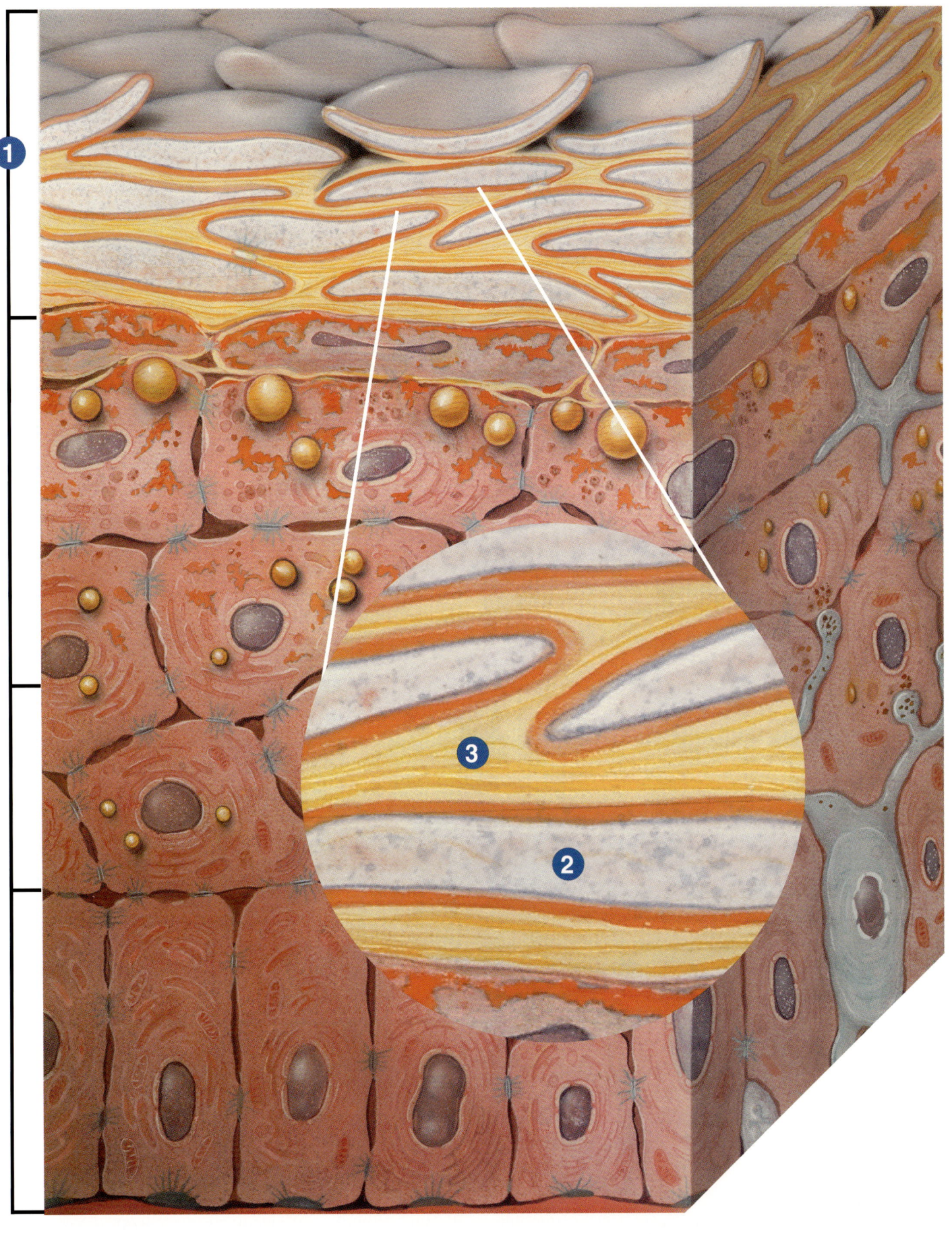

al carriage. Grooming behavior in normal dogs and excess licking in pruritic dogs may then seed the skin from these mucous membranes.

Staphylococcus intermedius AND OTHER CANINE CUTANEOUS PATHOGENS

Coagulase-positive staphylococci have long been considered the primary canine cutaneous bacterial pathogen.[3,25] Appropriate classification of this bacterium as S. intermedius, a species separate and distinct from the human pathogen S. aureus, was accomplished shortly thereafter.[11,12,26-29] This bacterium was previously believed to be a separate strain of S. aureus and more closely related to the primary human skin pathogen.[30]

Pure cultures of coagulase-positive S. intermedius are grown from most pustules or draining tracts in dogs with pyoderma.[3-7] Under most circumstances, when gram-negative bacteria such as Proteus, Pseudomonas, or Escherichia coli are cultured from canine pyoderma, they are grown in conjunction with S. intermedius from an open lesion. If gram-negative bacteria are isolated from a pyoderma without concomitant isolation of S. intermedius, the technique used and the results obtained should be questioned. S. intermedius infection creates a tissue milieu conducive to secondary gram-negative bacterial invasion.[4,5,7]

Various protein products and toxins considered to be virulence factors are elaborated by strains of staphylococci and relate to the degree of pathogenicity in humans. Similar data have not been elucidated for canine staphylococcal infections. This fact is underscored by the frequent inability to predict the course of bacterial skin disease in the dog. Protein A has been identified in the dog.[31-33] It is elaborated by some staphylococci that can prevent specific antibody access, prematurely trigger the complement cascade, and act as a chemoattractant for neutrophils. Protein A is known to be responsible for much of the inflammatory response to staphylococci in humans; however, its role in canine pyoderma is unknown. Leucocidin, hemolysins, epidermolytic toxin, and other soluble products may be important in the host response to pyoderma.[34] A hypersensitivity to staphylococcal antigens may promote the penetration of staphylococcal antigens by affecting epidermal permeability barriers.[35,36] When examined, virulence factors compar-

> *S. intermedius* infection creates a tissue milieu conducive to secondary gram-negative bacterial invasion.

ing S. intermedius isolates from normal dogs to those in dogs with pyoderma have indicated no clear differences in toxin profiles, SDS-PAGE (sodium dodecyl sulfate-polyacrylamide gel electrophoresis) of exoproteins, or immunoblotting of concentrated extracellular proteins.[37-39] Based on current knowledge, host rather than virulence factors appear to be more important in determining the outcome of cases of canine pyoderma.

ALTERATIONS IN MICROFLORA SEEN WITH SKIN DISEASE

The factors that promote the proliferation of S. intermedius on skin and lead to the likelihood of pyoderma are poorly understood. However, a number of studies indicate that dogs with various other skin diseases are more likely to develop secondary pyoderma.

Not surprisingly, it has been shown that dogs with pyoderma do not have a normal bacterial flora colonizing regions of the body without evident pyoderma. In a study of dogs with furunculosis, normal-appearing areas of the skin demonstrated an increase in both the frequency and the intensity of pathogenic staphylococcal colonization.[40] Recent work has corroborated that the populations of pathogenic coagulase-positive staphylococci increase on nonlesional skin of dogs with pyoderma.[24,36]

Dogs with cornification abnormalities have a shift in the balance of bacterial species colonizing the skin such that coagulase-positive staphylococci predominate.[9,41] This higher-than-normal frequency and density of pathogenic staphylococci was noted on nonlesional and lesional skin; however, bacterial counts were significantly higher in lesional skin. Consequently, it is not surprising that clinicians have noted an increased frequency of pyoderma in seborrheic dogs since a marked quantitative and qualitative shift to a pathogenic resident population has occurred. Simultaneous work by Kristensen and Krogh corroborated these findings and added that a similar shift in both the frequency and the intensity of staphylococcal colonization also was present in a group of dogs with atopic, contact, and seborrheic dermatitis.[42]

When long-term changes occur in the cutaneous microenvironment due to chronic allergic diseases, proliferation of S. intermedius may lead to recurrent pyoderma.[35,36,43] A recent study comparing the carriage of S. intermedius between normal dogs and asymptomatic atopic dogs receiving low-dose alternate-day corticosteroids revealed no overall differences. These data imply that either the inflammation of allergic diseases or the epidermal proliferation associated with underlying inflammation may predispose dogs to secondary pyoderma.[44]

ZOONOTIC POTENTIAL OF CANINE SKIN PATHOGENS

The documentation of S. intermedius as a separate and distinct species from S. aureus partially explains why humans with a normally functioning immune system do not seem to be at great risk for canine staphylococcal skin or wound infections (with the exception of canine bite wounds). Under usual circumstances, owners of dogs with staphylococcal pyoderma are not at risk for zoonotic bacterial infection. A recent review article discussing the zoonotic potential of pets owned by immunocompromised persons did not address concerns associated with canine skin pathogens.[45] However, in a previous study, S. intermedius was isolated from the gingiva of 39% of 135 dogs. When previously collected coagulase-positive *Staphylococcus* from infected, canine-inflicted human wounds were reanalyzed, 21% of 14 strains isolated were found to be S. intermedius.[46] These findings have been corroborated by others.[47] Consequently, a dog with severe suppurating pyoderma would be of concern in a household with an immunocompromised person.

Additional data of public health interest have been published in the recent literature. One previously unconsidered source of resistance to antibiotics is the transfer of resistance plasmids from bacteria carried by domesticated animals to bacteria of pathogenic importance in humans such as S. aureus.[48–50] Resistance plasmids from infections in humans could be transferred to canine pathogens in a similar manner. Enterotoxins from S. intermedius acting as bacterial super-antigens have been shown to cause naturally occurring staphylococcal food poisoning in humans. However, to date, the strains implicated have not been shown to be genetically similar to strains isolated from domesticated animals.[51] Quantitative analysis of enterotoxin production from S. intermedius has been shown to be one tenth to one hundredth that of enterotoxin production from S. aureus, reducing the likelihood of animal contamination that leads to staphylococcal food poisoning in humans.[50]

> One previously unconsidered source of resistance to antibiotics is the transfer of resistance plasmids from bacteria carried by domesticated animals to bacteria of pathogenic importance in humans such as S. aureus.

REFERENCES

1. Lloyd DH, Garthwaite G: Epidermal structure and surface topography of canine skin. *Res Vet Sci* 33:99–104, 1982.
2. Mason IS, Lloyd DH: Scanning electron microscopical studies of the living epidermis and stratum corneum of dogs, in Ihrke PJ, Mason IS, White SD (eds): *Advances in Veterinary Dermatology*, vol 2. Oxford, Pergamon, 1993, pp 131–139.
3. Ihrke PJ, Halliwell REW, Deubler MJ: Canine pyoderma, in Kirk RW (ed): *Current Veterinary Therapy VI*. Philadelphia, WB Saunders, 1976, pp 513–519.
4. Ihrke PJ: An overview of bacterial skin disease in the dog. *Br Vet J* 433: 112–118, 1987.
5. Ihrke PJ: Bacterial infections of the skin, in Greene CE (ed): *Infectious Diseases of the Dog and Cat*. Philadelphia, WB Saunders, 1990, pp 72–79.
6. Mason IS: Canine pyoderma. *J Small Anim Pract* 32:381–386, 1991.
7. Scott DW, Miller WH, Griffin CE: *Muller & Kirk's Small Animal Dermatology*, ed 5. Philadelphia, WB Saunders, 1995, pp 294–296.
8. Ihrke PJ, Schwartzman RM, McGinley K, et al: Microbiology of normal and seborrheic canine skin. *Am J Vet Res* 39:1487–1489, 1978.
9. Krogh HV, Kristensen S: A study of skin diseases of dogs and cats—II. Microflora of the normal skin of dogs and cats. *Nord Vet Med* 28:459–463, 1976.
10. Harvey RG, Noble WC, Lloyd DH: Distribution of propionibacteria on dogs: A preliminary report of the findings on 11 dogs. *J Small Anim Pract* 34:80–84, 1993.
11. Hajek V, Marsalek E: Evaluation of classificatory criteria for staphylococci, in Jeljaszewicz J (ed): Proceedings of the Third International Symposium of Staphylococci and Staphylococcal Infections, 1975, pp 11–21.
12. Hajek V: *Staphylococcus intermedius*, a new species isolated from animals. *Int J Syst Bacteriol* 26(Oct):401–408, 1976.
13. Hearst BR: Low incidence of staphylococcal dermatitides in animals with high incidence of *Staphylococcus aureus*. Part 2: Preliminary studies of dogs. *Vet Med Small Anim Clin* June:541–542, 1967.
14. White SD, Ihrke PJ, Stannard AA, et al: Occurrence of *Staphylococcus aureus* on the clinically normal canine hair coat. *Am J Vet Res* 44:332–334, 1983.
15. Kwochka KW: Qualitative and quantitative incidence of staphylococci on normal canine skin and haircoat: An investigation into the possibility of two different microbial populations. *Proc Am Acad Am Coll Vet Dermatol* 2:31, 1986.
16. Berg JN, Wendell DE, Vogelweid C, Fales WH: Identification of the major coagulase-positive *Staphylococcus* species of dogs as *Staphylococcus intermedius*. *Am J Vet Res* 45(7):1307–1309, 1984.
17. Allaker RP, Lloyd DH, Simpson AI: Occurrence of *Staphylococcus intermedius* on the hair and skin of normal dogs. *Res Vet Sci* 52:174–176, 1992.

18. Summers MM, Lynch PF, Black T: Hair as a reservoir of staphylococci. *J Clin Pathol* 18:13–15, 1965.
19. Noble WC: *Staphylococcus aureus* on the hair. *J Clin Pathol* 19:570–572, 1966.
20. McGinley KJ, Leyden JJ, Marples RR, Kligman AM: Quantitative microbiology of the scalp in nondandruff, dandruff, and seborrheic dermatitis. *J Invest Dermatol* 64:401–405, 1975.
21. Devriese LA, De Pelsmaecker K: The anal region as a main carrier site of *Staphylococcus intermedius* and *Streptococcus canis* in dogs. *Vet Rec* 121:302–303, 1987.
22. Allaker RP, Lloyd DH, Bailey RM: Population sizes and frequency of staphylococci at mucocutaneous sites on healthy dogs. *Vet Rec* 130:303–304, 1992.
23. Allaker RP, Jensen L, Lloyd DH, Lamport AI: Colonization of neonatal puppies by staphylococci. *Br Vet J* 148:523–528, 1992.
24. Lloyd DH, Allaker RP, Pattinson A: Carriage of *Staphylococcus intermedius* on the ventral abdomen of clinically normal dogs and those with pyoderma. *Vet Dermatol* 2(3/4):161–164, 1991.
25. Muller GH, Kirk RW: *Small Animal Dermatology*, ed 2. Philadelphia, WB Saunders, 1976, pp 223–230.
26. Phillips WE, Kloos WE: Identification of coagulase-positive *Staphylococcus intermedius* and *Staphylococcus hyicus* subsp. *hyicus* isolates from veterinary clinical specimens. *J Clin Microbiol* 14:671–673, 1981.
27. Biberstein EL, Jang SS, Hirsh DC: Species distribution of coagulase-positive staphylococci in animals. *J Clin Microbiol* 19:610–615, 1984.
28. Berg JN, Wendell DE, Vogelweid C, et al: Identification of the major coagulase-positive *Staphylococcus* sp. of dogs as *Staphylococcus intermedius*. *Am J Vet Res* 45:1307–1309, 1984.
29. Cox HU, Newman SS, Roy AF, Hoskins JD: Species of staphylococcus isolated from animal infections. *Cornell Vet* 74:124–135, 1984.
30. Live I: Differentiation of *Staphylococcus aureus* of human and of canine origins: Coagulation of human and of canine plasma, fibrinolysin activity, and serologic reaction. *Am J Vet Res* 33:385–391, 1972.
31. Cox HU, Schmeer N, Newman SS: Protein A in *Staphylococcus intermedius* isolates from dogs and cats. *Am J Vet Res* 47(9):1881–1884, 1986.
32. Fehrer-Sawyer SL: Identification and quantitation of protein A on canine *Staphylococcus intermedius*. *Proc Am Acad Coll Vet Dermatol* 2:13, 1986.
33. Greene RT, Lammler CH: Isolation and characterization of immunoglobulin binding proteins from *Staphylococcus intermedius* and *Staphylococcus hyicus*. *J Vet Med* 39:519–525, 1992.
34. Halliwell REW: Current therapy in recurrent pyoderma. *Proc Voorjarsdagen*, Amsterdam, 73, 1986.
35. Mason IS, Lloyd DH: The role of allergy in the development of canine pyoderma. *J Small Anim Pract* 30:216–218, 1989.
36. Mason IS: Hypersensitivity and the multiplication of staphylococci on canine skin (PhD thesis). London, University of London, 1990, pp 1–172.
37. Allaker RP, Lamport AI, Lloyd DH, Noble WC: Production of "virulence factors" by *Staphylococcus intermedius* from cases of canine pyoderma and healthy carriers. *Microbiol Ecol Health Dis* 4:169–173, 1991.
38. Allaker RP, Garrett N, Kent L, Noble WC, Lloyd DH: Characterisation of *Staphylococcus intermedius* isolates from canine pyoderma and from healthy carriers by SDS-PAGE of exoproteins, immunoblotting and restriction endonuclease digest analysis. *J Med Microbiol* 39:429–433, 1993.
39. Greene RT, Lammler CH: *Staphylococcus intermedius*: Current knowledge on a pathogen of veterinary importance. *J Vet Med* 40:206–214, 1993.
40. Quadros E: Furunculosis in dogs: Etiology, pathogenesis and treatment. *Acta Vet Scand* 52(Suppl):1–114, 1974.
41. Horwitz LN, Ihrke PJ: Canine seborrhea, in Kirk RW (ed): *Current Veterinary Therapy VI*. Philadelphia, WB Saunders, 1976, pp 519–524.
42. Kristensen S, Krogh HV: A study of skin diseases in dogs and cats—III. Microflora of the skin of dogs with chronic eczema. *Nord Vet Med* 30:223–230, 1978.
43. McEwan NA: Bacterial adherence to canine corneocytes, in Von Tscharner C, Halliwell REW (eds): *Advances in Veterinary Dermatology*, vol 1. London, Baillière Tindall, 1990, p 454.
44. Harvey RG, Noble WC: A temporal study comparing the carriage of *Staphylococcus intermedius* on normal dogs with atopic dogs in clinical remission. *Vet Dermatol* 5(1):21–25, 1994.
45. Angulo FJ, Glaser CA, Jurnaek DD, et al: Caring for pets of immunocompromised persons. *JAVMA* 205(12):1711–1718, 1994.
46. Talan DA, Staatz D, Staatz A, et al: *Staphylococcus intermedius* in canine gingiva and canine-inflicted human wound infections: Laboratory characterizations of a newly recognized zoonotic pathogen. *J Clin Microbiol* 27(1):78–81, 1989.
47. Lee J: *Staphylococcus intermedius* isolated from dog-bite wounds. *J Infect* 29:118, 1994.
48. Davies M, Stewart PR: Transferable drug resistance in man and animals: Genetic relationship between R-plasmids in enteric bacteria from man and domestic pets. *Aust Vet J* 54:507–512, 1978.
49. Forbes BA, Schaberg DR: Transfer of resistance plasmids from *Staphylococcus epidermidis* to *Staphylococcus aureus*: Evidence for conjugative exchange of resistance. *J Bacteriol* 153:627–634, 1983.
50. Naido J, Lloyd DH: Transmission of genes between staphylococci on skin, in Woodbine M (ed): *Antimicrobials in Agriculture*, Monograph 23. London, British Government Press, 1984, pp 285–292.
51. Khambaty FM, Bennett RW, Shah DB: Application of pulsed field gel electrophoresis to the epidemiological characterization of *Staphylococcus intermedius* implicated in a food-related outbreak. *Epidemiol Infect* 113:75–81, 1994.

Chapter 3

Canine Pyoderma—Susceptibility and the Host Response to Infection

SUSCEPTIBILITY TO INFECTION

Staphylococcus intermedius, the primary cutaneous bacterial pathogen responsible for causing the great majority of canine pyodermas, does not possess the requisite virulence factors to be considered a potent pathogen for the normal dog.[1-3] Consequently, unless other virulence factors are identified, most bacterial infections seen in canine skin are probably associated with either underlying disease or host factors that favor the establishment of bacterial infection. Pyoderma has, by tradition, been classified as either primary or secondary to reflect the lack of identification or identification of underlying causes. As our knowledge of the condition has increased, the percentage of diagnoses of "primary pyoderma" has diminished whereas the percentage of diagnoses of "secondary pyoderma" has expanded.

The factors leading to the initiation of canine pyoderma are protean. Anatomic abnormalities such as skin folds can lead to bacterial overgrowth giving rise to intertrigo, commonly classified as a skin-fold pyoderma. Preexisting diseases such as ectoparasitism, cornification defects (seborrhea), allergy (atopic dermatitis, food allergy, and flea allergy dermatitis), and endocrinopathies such as hypothyroidism and Cushing's disease, frequently predispose dogs to the development of pyoderma[4-8] (Table 3-1). The potential for secondary pyoderma is best documented in dogs with cornification abnormalities and allergic diseases.[9-14] In addition, poor grooming, pruritus from any underlying disease, inflammation from any cause, and the injudicious use of corticosteroids contribute to the likelihood of secondary infection. Well-documented primary immunodeficiency as a cause of canine pyoderma is rare. Primary immunodeficiencies documented in the dog have been recently reviewed.[8] In contrast, acquired immunologic defects in the ability to fight bacterial infection are more common as exemplified by naturally occurring and acquired hyperglucocorticoidism, hypothyroidism, and demodicosis.

Once a pyoderma has been initiated, immunologic incompetence, coexisting disease, pruritus, inflammation, scar tissue formation, and improper initial therapy are all negative prognostic factors. The presence of pruritus or severe inflammation is often a marker of frustration as

TABLE 3-1
FACTORS LEADING TO THE DEVELOPMENT OF CANINE PYODERMA

- **ANATOMIC ABNORMALITIES**
  Skin folds

- **PREEXISTING DISEASES**
  Ectoparasitism
  Cornification defects
    Seborrhea
  Allergy
    Atopic dermatitis
    Food allergy
    Flea allergy dermatitis

- **ENDOCRINOPATHIES**
  Hypothyroidism
  Cushing's disease

these cases may be substantially more difficult to manage.[5,6,15]

Bacterial infections of the hair follicle are the single largest subgrouping of pyoderma. Dogs with inflammation, obstruction, atrophy, dysplasia, or degeneration of the hair follicles are predisposed to secondary pyoderma. Preexisting inflammation of the hair follicles that initiates a secondary pyoderma may be seen in conjunction with other infectious follicular diseases. Pyoderma secondary to demodicosis is common, whereas pyoderma secondary to dermatophytic infections of hair follicles apparently is rare. Pyoderma caused by underlying follicular inflammation and obstruction can be a sequela to generalized or localized defects in cornification. Thus, folliculitis and furunculosis is seen secondary to generalized seborrhea as well as to localized keratinization or cornification abnormalities such as schnauzer comedo syndrome and callus pyoderma. Pyoderma secondary to follicular abnormalities may even have marked breed predilections. For example, secondary superficial bacterial folliculitis or deep bacterial folliculitis and furunculosis is a prominent feature of sebaceous adenitis in the Akita and is rarely seen in other breeds at risk for sebaceous adenitis, such as the standard poodle. Pyoderma also may be seen secondary to congenital dysplastic diseases of the hair follicle, such as color dilution alopecia, black hair follicular dysplasia, and congenital hypotrichosis.

HOST RESPONSE TO INFECTION: BENEFICIAL AND DELETERIOUS

The initiation of a staphylococcal pyoderma in a susceptible dog involves a complex sequence of interactions between the bacteria and the dog (Figure 3-1). Entry of the bacteria, if successful, requires invasion and colonization of host tissues and evasion of host immunity. Successful invasion leads to tissue injury or some functional impairment.

Beneficial Host Response

Nonimmunologic host defense mechanisms that limit bacterial colonization and presumedly diminish the likelihood of localized infection becoming more generalized include desquamation of the stratum corneum from the epidermal surface and the hair follicles, the intercellular lipid-rich barrier between the cells of the stratum corneum, which provides a physical barrier to bacterial invasion, epithelial proliferation in response to tissue injury, and the antibacterial effect of inorganic salts found in sebum and sweat. These nonimmunologic host defense mechanisms may lead to unsuccessful entry of the bacteria. Resident bacterial competition is an additional fortuitous nonimmunologic, "nonhost" defense mechanism.

The immune response against extracellular cocci such as *S. intermedius* is directed toward eliminating the bacteria and neutralizing the effects of toxins produced by the bacteria. Immunologic host defense mechanisms of the skin, termed the *skin immune system* (SIS), include immunologically active proteins within the lipid-rich intercellular matrix, immunoglobulins within the basement membrane zone, and the cells of the immune system present in the epidermis and dermis.[16,17] The skin immune system coupled with regional lymphoid tissue are termed the *skin associated lymphoid tissue* (SALT).[17,18] Immunoglobulin A (IgA) and immunoglobulin G (IgG) have been identified within the intercellular barrier between the cells of the stratum corneum, and immunoglobulin M (IgM) has been found within the basement membrane zone.[19] The immunologically active cells within the epidermis and dermis comprising the skin immune system include Langerhans' cells, dermal dendrocytes, lymphocytes, mast cells, and the endothelial cells of postcapillary venules.[16–18]

Humoral immunity is classically described as providing primary defense against bacterial invasion. Immunogenic components of the bacteria such as polysaccharides from the bacterial cell wall directly stimulate B cells, which leads to a strong IgM response. Both extracellular cocci and soluble bacterial antigens are phagocytosed by various antigen-presenting cells.[20] Bone marrow–derived B lymphocytes differentiate into plasma cells that produce IgG, IgM, IgA, and immunoglobulin E (IgE). Helper T lymphocytes facilitate antibody production while suppressor T lymphocytes can suppress antibody production by modulating B lymphocyte function. IgM and IgG directed against bacterial surface antigens stimulate various effector mechanisms. Effector cells play an important role in eliminating antigen. IgG antibodies opsonize bacteria and enhance phagocytosis, and IgG and IgM neutralize bacterial toxins, preventing them from binding to target cells and activating the complement system, which leads to acute inflammation.

> Bacterial infections of the hair follicle are the single largest subgrouping of pyoderma.

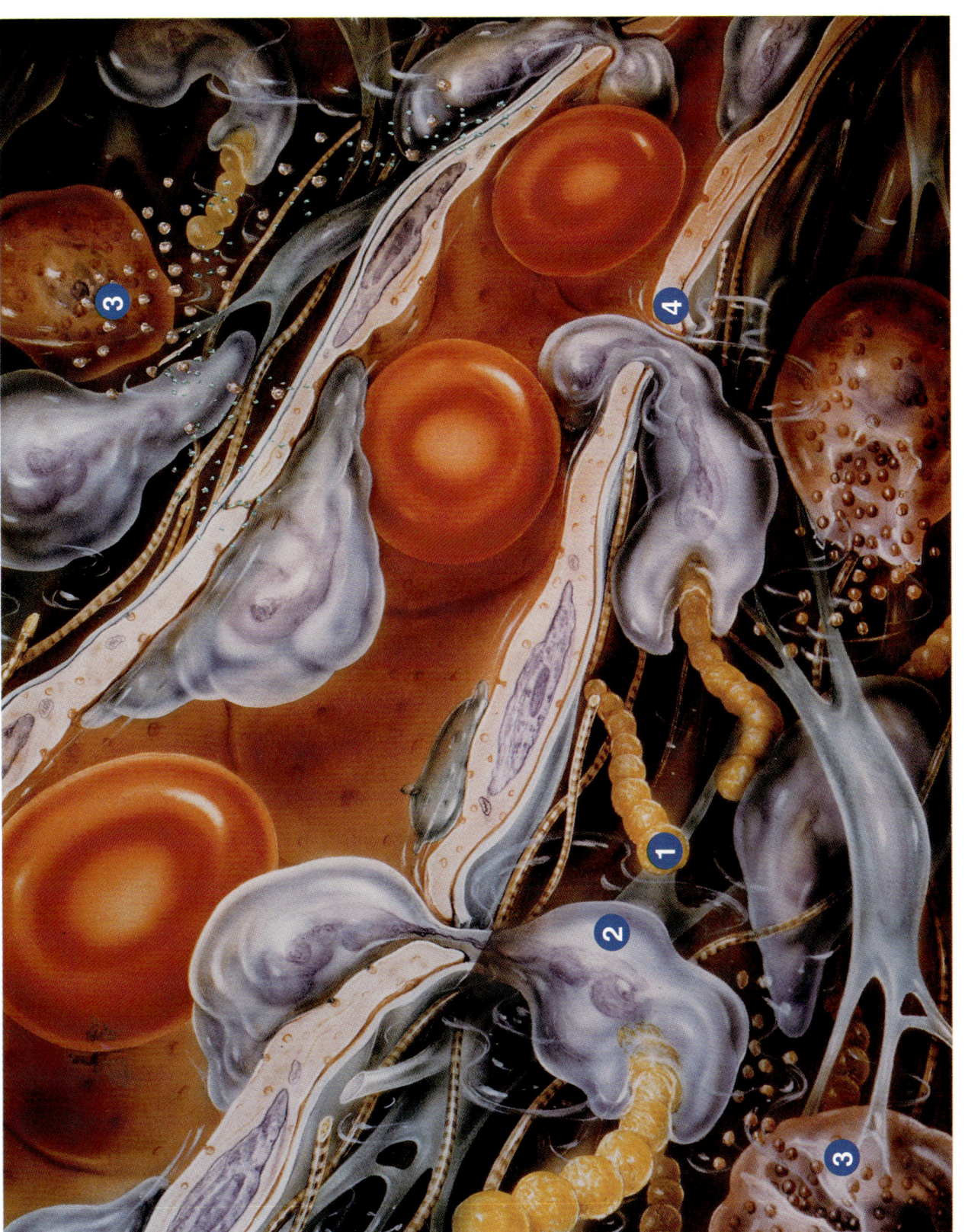

FIGURE 3-1 *Inflammation. The immune response against extracellular cocci such as Staphylococcus intermedius is directed toward eliminating the bacteria and neutralizing the effects of toxins produced by the bacteria. (1) Bacteria invade tissues and liberate toxins and other substances. (2) Neutrophils and macrophages phagocytize bacteria but also excrete numerous proteolytic enzymes and chemotactic and chemokinetic substances that attract more white cells. (3) Mast cells degranulate and liberate vasoactive amines. (4) The action of vasoactive substances leads to vasodilation and leakage of plasma and protein into tissue. (Courtesy of Bayer AG.)*

Deleterious Host Response

Host immunologic response to bacterial antigens may be deleterious as well as beneficial. Experimental and clinical evidence indicate that some dogs with chronic or recurrent pyoderma exhibit depression of lymphocyte blastogenesis during periods of active infection.[8,21-23] Recent experimental work by DeBoer adds that staphylococcal antigen and laboratory-prepared staphylococcal immune complex can modulate some inflammatory cell functions in vitro. Macrophage function was inhibited while neutrophil function was mildly stimulated.[24]

Some bacterial antigens are known to stimulate inappropriately large numbers of helper T lymphocytes. These exceptionally potent antigens have been termed *super-antigens*. The enterotoxin that produces staphylococcal food poisoning and the related toxin that produces toxic shock syndrome are examples of super-antigens.[20,25] Recently, *S. aureus* cultured from the lesions of humans with atopic dermatitis has been shown to produce super-antigens. Super-antigen binding to surface receptors on macrophages is known to lead to the release of tumor necrosis factor α and interleukin 6. T lymphocyte activation by staphylococcal super-antigens also may lead to marked cytokine release. Together, these two mechanisms may explain the marked clinical exacerbation of the lesions of atopic dermatitis by secondary staphylococcal colonization.[26] Similar pathogenic mechanisms may explain the troublesome nature of pyoderma secondary to atopic dermatitis in dogs. Fadok and Edwards have speculated that bacterial super-antigens may play a role in the severe inflammation evident with some canine pyoderma.[27] These super-antigens could play a role in the marked inflammation and pruritus seen with certain subgroups of canine pyoderma.

In humans, bacterial endotoxins and super-antigens may contribute to the development of autoimmunity.[20] It is interesting to speculate that a similar process might be occurring in the dog because pyoderma is seen more commonly in the dog than in any other species studied, and the relative frequency of autoimmune skin diseases in the dog is much higher than that seen in humans.

Bacterial hypersensitivity has long been hypothesized to be an initiator or complicating and perpetuating feature of recurrent canine pyoderma[28,29] and has been proven to occur in humans in association with hyperimmunoglobulin E syndrome and, more commonly, in humans with atopic dermatitis.[30-32] Preliminary data by Halliwell indicated higher levels of antistaphylococcal IgE in dogs with recurrent pyoderma and erythematous spreading lesions.[33] A larger study by Morales and others substantiated an association among antistaphylococcal antibodies and various subgroups of canine pyoderma.[34] Dogs with idiopathic recurrent superficial pyoderma and dogs with recurrent pyoderma secondary to atopy had significantly higher mean levels of serum antistaphylococcal IgE than did normal control dogs, dogs with nonrecurrent pyoderma, and dogs with idiopathic recurrent deep pyoderma. The authors speculate that "cutaneous mast cell–bound antistaphylococcal IgE may trigger the release of inflammatory mediators in the presence of staphylococcal antigens."[34] Mediator release may lead to inflammation, additional mediator release, clinical signs, and locally impaired neutrophil chemotaxis. Research by Mason and Lloyd indicates that mast cell degranulation can initiate enhanced epidermal permeability to bacterial antigens in atopic dogs.[12,13] These data present an appealing scenario to explain recurrent pyoderma in atopic dogs. Morales and others stated in their report that dogs with idiopathic recurrent superficial pyoderma had been intradermally skin tested to rule out atopy.[34] These dogs could have been skin test–negative atopic dogs and still fulfilled the criteria of Willemse for canine atopy.[35]

In the previously mentioned study by Morales and others, all groups of dogs with prior pyoderma had significantly higher mean serum antistaphylococcal IgG levels than did normal dogs.[34] The elevated IgG response in dogs with previous pyoderma may simply represent a possibly helpful host response related to the magnitude and duration of previous infections.

REFERENCES

1. Allaker RP, Lamport AI, Lloyd DH, Noble WC: Production of "virulence factors" by *Staphylococcus intermedius* from cases of canine pyoderma and healthy carriers. Microbiol Ecol Health Dis 4:169–173, 1991.
2. Allaker RP, Garrett N, Kent L, et al: Characterization of *Staphylococcus*

intermedius isolates from canine pyoderma and from healthy carriers by SDS-PAGE of exoproteins, immunoblotting and restriction endonuclease digest analysis. *J Med Microbiol* 39:429–433, 1993.
3. Greene RT, Lammler CH: *Staphylococcus intermedius*: Current knowledge on a pathogen of veterinary importance. *J Vet Med* 40:206–214, 1993.
4. Ihrke PJ, Halliwell REW, Deubler MJ: Canine pyoderma, in Kirk RW (ed): *Current Veterinary Therapy VI*. Philadelphia, WB Saunders, 1976, pp 513–519.
5. Ihrke PJ: An overview of bacterial skin disease in the dog. *Br Vet J* 433:112–118, 1987.
6. Ihrke PJ: Bacterial infections of the skin, in: Greene CE (ed): *Infectious Diseases of the Dog and Cat*. Philadelphia, WB Saunders, 1990, pp 72–79.
7. Mason IS: Canine pyoderma. *J Small Anim Pract* 32:381–386, 1991.
8. Scott DW, Miller WH, Griffin CE: *Muller & Kirk's Small Animal Dermatology*, ed 5. Philadelphia, WB Saunders, 1995, pp 279–328.
9. Horwitz LN, Ihrke PJ: Canine seborrhea, in Kirk RW (ed): *Current Veterinary Therapy VI*. Philadelphia, WB Saunders, 1976, pp 519–524.
10. Ihrke PJ, Schwartzman RM, McGinley K, et al: Microbiology of normal and seborrheic canine skin. *Am J Vet Res* 39:1487–1489, 1978.
11. Kristensen S, Krogh HV: A study of skin diseases in dogs and cats—III. Microflora of the skin of dogs with chronic eczema. *Nord Vet Med* 30:223–230, 1978.
12. Mason IS, Lloyd DH: The role of allergy in the development of canine pyoderma. *J Small Anim Pract* 30:216–218, 1989.
13. Mason IS: Hypersensitivity and the multiplication of staphylococci on canine skin (PhD thesis). London, University of London, 1990, pp 1–172.
14. Harvey RG, Noble WC: A temporal study comparing the carriage of *Staphylococcus intermedius* on normal dogs with atopic dogs in clinical remission. *Vet Dermatol* 5(1):21–25, 1994.
15. Gross TL, Ihrke PJ, Walder EJ: *Veterinary Dermatopathology: A Macroscopic and Microscopic Evaluation of Canine and Feline Skin Disease*. St. Louis, Mosby–Year Book, 1992, pp 10–14, 231–238, 252–257.
16. Stingl G, Tschachler E, Groh V, Wolff K: The immune functions of epidermal cells, in Norris DA (ed): *Immune Mechanisms in Cutaneous Disease*. New York, Marcel Dekker, 1989, pp 3–72.
17. Yager JA: The skin as an immunologic organ, in Ihrke PJ, Mason IS, White SD (eds): *Advances in Veterinary Dermatology*, vol 2. Oxford, Pergamon Press, 1993, pp 3–31.
18. Streilen JW: Skin-associated lymphoid tissue, in Norris DA (ed): *Immune Mechanisms in Cutaneous Disease*. New York, Marcel Dekker, 1989, pp 73–96.
19. Garthwaite G, Lloyd DH, Thomsett LR: The location of immunoglobulins and complement (C3) at the surface and within the skin of dogs. *J Comp Pathol* 93:185–193, 1983.
20. Abbas AK, Lichtman AH, Pober JS: *Cellular and Molecular Immunology*, ed 2. Philadelphia, WB Saunders, 1994, pp 320–336.
21. Barta O, Waltman C, Oyekan PP, et al: Lymphocyte transformation suppression caused by pyoderma—Failure to demonstrate it in uncomplicated demodectic mange. *Comp Immunol Microbiol Infect Dis* 6:9–17, 1983.
22. Barta O: Immunomodulatory effect of serum on lymphocytes—Consequences for the study of immunostimulants *in vitro* and *in vivo*. *Comp Immunol Microbiol Infect Dis* 9:193–203, 1986.
23. Ihrke PJ: Antibacterial therapy in dermatology, in Kirk RW (ed): *Current Veterinary Therapy IX*. Philadelphia, WB Saunders, 1985, pp 566–571.
24. DeBoer DJ: Immunomodulatory effects of staphylococcal antigen and antigen-antibody complexes on canine mononuclear and polymorphonuclear leukocytes. *Am J Vet Res* 55(12):1690–1696, 1994.
25. Marrack P, Kapplier J: The staphylococcal enterotoxins and their relatives. *Science* 248:705–711, 1990.
26. McFadden JP, Noble WC, Camp RDR: Superantigenic exotoxin-secreting potential of staphylococci isolated from atopic eczematous skin. *Br J Dermatol* 128:631–632, 1993.
27. Fadok VA, Edwards MD: Advances in immunology. Proceedings of the Annual Meeting of the American Academy/College of Veterinary Dermatology (Resident Training Session Supplement), Santa Fe, New Mexico, 1995, pp 1–14.
28. Baker E: Staphylococcal disease. *Vet Clin North Am Small Anim Pract*. 4:107–117, 1974.
29. Scott DW, MacDonald JM, Schultz RD: Staphylococcal hypersensitivity in the dog. *JAAHA* 14:766–779, 1978.
30. Schopfer K, Baerlocher K, Price P, et al: Staphylococcal IgE antibodies, hyperimmunoglobulinemia E and *Staphylococcus aureus* infections. *N Engl J Med* 300:835–838, 1979.
31. Abramson JS, Dahl MV, Walsh G, et al: Antistaphylococcal IgE in patients with atopic dermatitis. *J Am Acad Dermatol* 7:105–110, 1982.
32. Friedman SJ, Schroeter AL, Homburger HA: IgE antibodies to *Staphylococcus aureus*. Prevalence in patients with atopic dermatitis. *Arch Dermatol* 1221:869–872, 1985.
33. Halliwell REW: Levels of IgE and IgG antibodies to staphylococcal antigens in normal dogs and in dogs with recurrent pyoderma. Proceedings American Academy/College of Veterinary Dermatology Annual Meeting, Phoenix, Arizona, 1987, p 5.
34. Morales CA, Schultz KT, DeBoer DJ: Antistaphylococcal antibodies in dogs with recurrent staphylococcal pyoderma. *Vet Immunol Immunopathol* 42:137–147, 1994.
35. Willemse T: Atopic skin disease: A review and a reconsideration of diagnostic criteria. *J Small Anim Pract* 27:771–778, 1986.

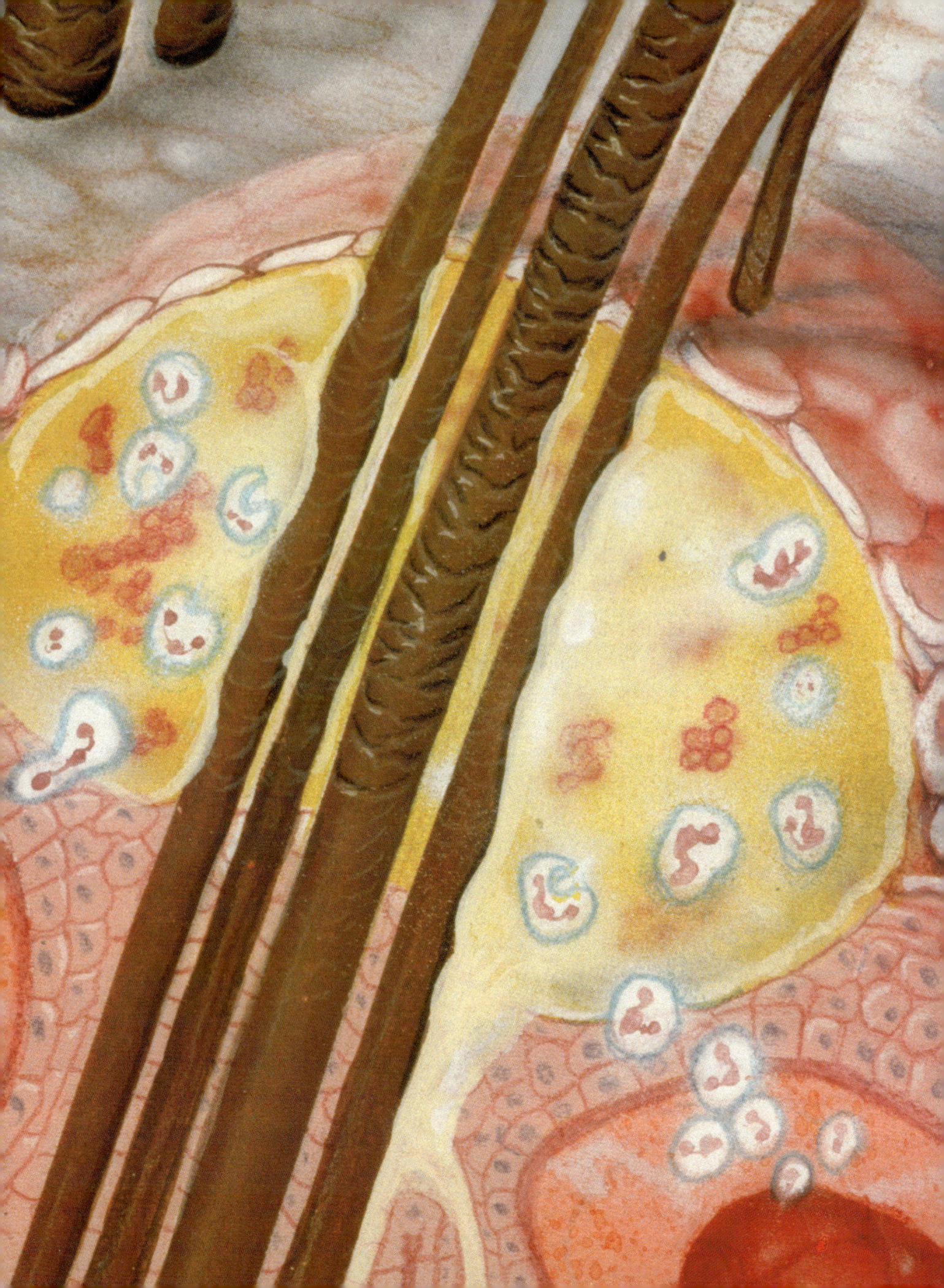

Chapter 4

Classification of Canine Pyoderma

Canine pyoderma has been classified or categorized based on various criteria. Anatomic site of infection (pressure-point pyoderma), the causative agent isolated (staphylococcal pyoderma), and the presence or absence of an identifiable underlying cause (primary versus secondary pyoderma) were used initially to categorize bacterial infections of canine skin.[1,2] Classification based on depth of bacterial involvement in the skin and the histologic site of infection were initially proposed two decades ago.[3] Since then, this classification scheme, with various modifications, has become the established method of classifying canine pyoderma.[4-15]

Classification based on depth of bacterial involvement is most useful clinically because clinical information referable to diagnosis, likelihood of underlying disease, prognosis, and response to therapy correlate with depth of infection. In general, the deeper the level of inflammation, the more likely underlying causes are present and the more aggressive the clinician must be both diagnostically and therapeutically.[7,10] Using depth of bacterial involvement and the histologic site of infection as criteria for classification, canine pyoderma may be subdivided as surface, superficial, and deep (Table 4-1).

SURFACE PYODERMA

The term *surface pyoderma* is applied to very superficial erosions of the skin. Although pathogenic bacteria (predominantly *Staphylococcus intermedius*) can be cultured routinely from these lesions and certainly contribute to inflammation and morbidity, bacterial involvement is secondary. Pyotraumatic dermatitis (acute moist dermatitis and hot spots), intertrigo (skin-fold pyoderma and skin-fold dermatitis) and mucocutaneous pyoderma can be classified as surface pyoderma. Pyotraumatic dermatitis develops as a sequela to underlying allergic skin disease

TABLE 4-1
CLASSIFICATION OF BACTERIAL INFECTION OF THE SKIN BASED ON DEPTH OF INFECTION

- **SURFACE PYODERMA**
  Pyotraumatic dermatitis (acute moist dermatitis and hot spots)
  Intertrigo (skin-fold pyoderma)
     Lip-fold intertrigo
     Facial-fold intertrigo
     Vulvar-fold intertrigo
     Tail-fold intertrigo
     Obesity-fold intertrigo
  Mucocutaneous pyoderma

- **SUPERFICIAL PYODERMA**
  Impetigo (puppy pyoderma)
  Superficial folliculitis*
  Superficial spreading pyoderma*

- **DEEP PYODERMA**
  Deep folliculitis and furunculosis
     Pyotraumatic folliculitis*
     Muzzle folliculitis and furunculosis (canine acne)
     Pedal folliculitis and furunculosis*
     Callus pyoderma (pressure-point pyoderma)
     German shepherd dog pyoderma*
  Cellulitis (secondary to demodicosis or immunologic incompetence)*

- **DISEASES FORMERLY CLASSIFIED AS PYODERMA**
  Juvenile sterile granulomatous dermatitis and lymphadenitis (juvenile cellulitis, puppy strangles, juvenile "pyoderma")
  Hidradenitis suppurativa (most were probably bullous pemphigoid or ulcerative dermatosis of the Shetland sheepdog and collie)

*Indicates subgroups of superficial and deep pyoderma where recurrence or recrudescence is more common.

TABLE 4-2
DIFFERENTIAL DIAGNOSIS OF CANINE PYODERMA

■ **SURFACE PYODERMA**

Pyotraumatic dermatitis (acute moist dermatitis and hot spots)
Pyotraumatic folliculitis, demodicosis, neoplasia—especially sweat gland adenocarcinoma, cutaneous metastasis, fixed drug eruption, early necrotizing form of idiopathic nodular panniculitis, early localized vasculitis, focal *Malassezia* dermatitis, and candidiasis

Intertrigo (skin-fold pyoderma)
Lip-fold intertrigo
  Localized demodicosis, fixed drug eruption, superficial necrolytic dermatitis with or without *Malassezia* dermatitis or candidiasis, zinc-responsive dermatosis, muzzle folliculitis and furunculosis (canine acne), localized pemphigus foliaceus, early pemphigus vulgaris, early bullous pemphigoid

Facial-fold intertrigo
  Localized demodicosis, *Malassezia* dermatitis, dermatophytosis

Vulvar-fold intertrigo
  Urinary tract infection with self-trauma, ulcerative dermatosis of the Shetland sheepdog and collie, drug eruption, canine familial dermatomyositis, pemphigus vulgaris, bullous pemphigoid

Tail-fold intertrigo
  Flea allergy dermatitis

Obesity-fold intertrigo
  Malassezia dermatitis

Mucocutaneous pyoderma
Lip-fold intertrigo, localized demodicosis, early discoid lupus erythematosus, zinc-responsive dermatosis, generic dog food skin disease, muzzle folliculitis and furunculosis (canine acne)

■ **SUPERFICIAL PYODERMA**

Impetigo (puppy pyoderma)
Early flea allergy dermatitis, superficial folliculitis

Superficial folliculitis
Superficial spreading pyoderma, flea allergy dermatitis, demodicosis, pemphigus foliaceus, sarcoptic acariasis, severe impetigo, drug eruption, erythema multiforme, seborrheic dermatitis, sterile eosinophilic pustulosis

Superficial spreading pyoderma
Superficial folliculitis, pemphigus foliaceus, erythema multiforme, sterile eosinophilic pustulosis

■ **DEEP PYODERMA**

Deep folliculitis and furunculosis
Demodicosis, subcutaneous and deep mycoses, severe maladapted dermatophytosis, sterile granuloma/pyogranuloma, histiocytosis, idiopathic nodular panniculitis, juvenile sterile granulomatous dermatitis and lymphadenitis, vasculitis

Pyotraumatic folliculitis
  Pyotraumatic dermatitis, demodicosis, neoplasia—especially sweat gland adenocarcinoma, cutaneous metastasis, fixed drug eruption, early necrotizing form of idiopathic nodular panniculitis, early localized vasculitis, focal *Malassezia* dermatitis, and candidiasis

Muzzle folliculitis and furunculosis (canine acne)
  Localized demodicosis, early juvenile sterile granulomatous dermatitis and lymphadenitis

Pedal folliculitis and furunculosis
  Demodicosis, dermatophytosis, subcutaneous and deep mycoses, opportunistic fungal diseases, *Pelodera* dermatitis

Callus pyoderma (pressure-point pyoderma)
  Acral lick dermatitis, generic dog food skin disease, focal actinic comedones

German shepherd dog pyoderma
  Demodicosis with secondary deep pyoderma, subcutaneous and deep mycosis, opportunistic fungal diseases

Cellulitis (with or without demodicosis)
Juvenile cellulitis, subcutaneous and deep mycosis, German shepherd dog pyoderma, sterile granuloma/pyogranuloma, idiopathic liquefying panniculitis

coupled with self-trauma. Flea allergy dermatitis is the most common underlying cause. Intertrigo is seen in conjunction with friction, poor drainage, and maceration at sites of skin folding. Intertrigo can be further subdivided based on the affected anatomic site. Lip-fold intertrigo, facial-fold intertrigo, and tail-fold intertrigo have marked breed predilections based on specific anatomic abnormalities considered as breed standards. Generalized fold intertrigo is seen in the Chinese shar-pei. Vulvar-fold intertrigo and obesity-fold intertrigo are associated with acquired anatomic abnormalities. Mucocutaneous pyoderma is an infection of unknown etiology that predominantly involves the lips and perioral skin. It may be present alone or coexist with lip-fold intertrigo.[12,16] Dogs with surface pyoderma are rarely presented as either a major diagnostic or therapeutic problem and constitute a minority of the cases of skin disease classified as pyoderma.

SUPERFICIAL PYODERMA

Superficial folliculitis is a large, pleomorphic subgrouping of pyoderma. Superficial pyodermas, the most common canine bacterial skin diseases, are among the most common canine dermatoses. The term *impetigo* is used to describe nonfollicular bacterial microabscessation involving the superficial layers of the epidermis. Superficial folliculitis involves the ostial portion of the hair follicle and is the single most common category of bacterial skin disease in the dog. Dogs with impetigo and superficial folliculitis are often presented as diagnostic challenges because pustules rupture easily and lead to less diagnostic crusted papules. A visually distinctive clinical subset of superficial pyoderma termed *superficial spreading pyoderma* is characterized by centrifugally progressive erythema and expanding peripheral epidermal collarettes. These lesions may be seen alone or, more commonly, in conjunction with superficial folliculitis.[12,17]

DEEP PYODERMA

In deep pyoderma, infection from the distal portion of the hair follicle may extend beneath and beyond the confines of the hair follicle. Follicular rupture may lead to a granulomatous tissue response. Deep pyoderma is much less common than superficial pyoderma and may be subdivided further into deep folliculitis and furunculosis and cellulitis. Although deep folliculitis remains within the confines of the hair follicles, follicular rupture with attendant foreign body granulomatous response is seen in furunculosis. Multiple subgroups are named based on the anatomic site of involvement. The term *cellulitis* implies that infection has become confluent, involving the dermis and the subjacent panniculus. Sepsis is a frequent sequela to this uncommon deep infection and is seen most often in conjunction with generalized demodicosis. Diagnosis of deep pyoderma may be less difficult than with superficial pyoderma, but therapy is often problematic.

OVERVIEW OF DIAGNOSTIC DIFFERENTIALS

A detailed discussion of all the diagnostic differentials of each subgroup of canine pyoderma is beyond the scope of this manual. Important diagnostic differentials, presented in approximate order of importance, are listed in Table 4-2. In addition, the reader is referred to Chapters 6, 7, and 8, where major diagnostic differentials are discussed under each disease heading.

REFERENCES

1. Kral F, Novak BJ: *Veterinary Dermatology*. Philadelphia, JB Lippincott, 1953, pp viii–ix.
2. Muller GH, Kirk RW: *Small Animal Dermatology*. Philadelphia, WB Saunders, 1976, pp 223–230.
3. Ihrke PJ, Halliwell REW, Deubler MJ: Canine pyoderma, in Kirk RW (ed): *Current Veterinary Therapy VI*. Philadelphia, WB Saunders, 1976, pp 513–519.
4. Ihrke PJ: The management of canine pyodermas, in Kirk RW (ed): *Current Veterinary Therapy VIII*. Philadelphia, WB Saunders, 1983, pp 505–517.
5. Ihrke PJ: Antibacterial therapy in dermatology, in Kirk RW (ed): *Current Veterinary Therapy IX*. Philadelphia, WB Saunders, 1985, pp 566–571.
6. Grant DI: *Skin Diseases in the Dog and Cat*. Oxford, Blackwell Scientific Publications, 1986, p 8.
7. Ihrke PJ: An overview of bacterial skin disease in the dog. *Br Vet J* 433:112–118, 1987.
8. White SD, Ihrke PJ: Pyoderma, in Nesbitt GH (ed): *Dermatology—Contemporary Issues in Small Animal Practice*. New York, Churchill Livingstone, 1987, pp 95–121.
9. Fourrier P, Carlotti D, Magnol J-P, et al: Les pyodermites du chien. *Prat Med Chirurg Animal Compag* 23(6):1–539, 1988.
10. Ihrke PJ: Bacterial infections of the skin, in Greene CE (ed): *Infectious Diseases of the Dog and Cat*. Philadelphia, WB Saunders, 1990, pp 72–79.
11. Mason IS: Canine pyoderma. *J Small Anim Pract* 32:381–386, 1991.
12. Gross TL, Ihrke PJ, Walder EJ: *Veterinary Dermatopathology: A Macroscopic and Microscopic Evaluation of Canine and Feline Skin Disease*. St. Louis, Mosby–Year Book, 1992, pp 10–14, 238–240, 252–255.
13. Kwochka KW: Recurrent pyoderma, in Griffin CE, Kwochka KW, Macdonald JM (eds): *Current Veterinary Dermatology*. St. Louis, Mosby–Year Book, 1993, pp 3–21.
14. Hill PB, Moriella KA: Canine pyoderma. *JAVMA* 204:334–340, 1994.
15. Scott DW, Miller WH, Griffin CE: *Muller & Kirk's Small Animal Dermatology*, ed 5. Philadelphia, WB Saunders, 1995, pp 61–66.
16. Ihrke PJ, Gross TL: Canine mucocutaneous pyoderma, in Bonagura JD (ed): *Kirk's Current Veterinary Therapy XII*. Philadelphia, WB Saunders, 1995, pp 618–619.
17. Ihrke PJ, Gross TL: Clinico-pathologic conferences in dermatology—#1: Superficial spreading pyoderma. *Vet Dermatol* 4(1):33–36, 1994.

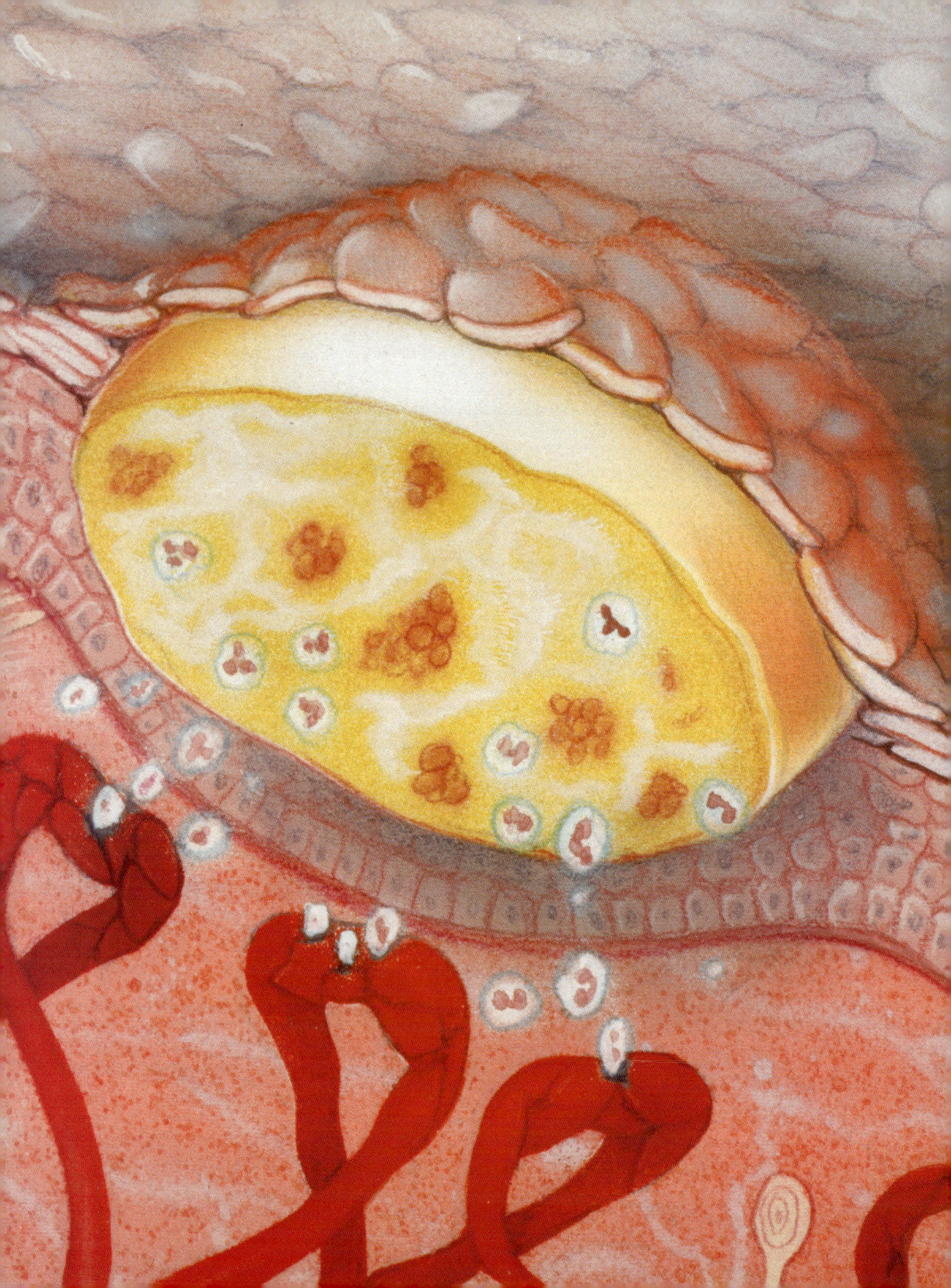

Chapter 5

General Clinical Findings

Dermatology has a singular advantage over many other medical specialty disciplines in that the gross pathology of the affected organ is visible and readily available for careful visual inspection and palpation. A wide variety of skin lesions, both primary and secondary, occur in canine pyoderma. Excellent lighting is essential for a proper physical examination of the skin. A lighted hand lens is additionally beneficial. If lesions occur in densely haired skin, clinical findings may be clarified by clipping the overlying hair from an affected area.

PRIMARY SKIN LESIONS

Erythematous **papules** and **pustules** are the most common primary skin lesions seen in most superficial and some deep pyodermas. Papules, which are circumscribed solid elevations of the skin, usually form in groups. As infection and resultant inflammation proceed, pus accumulates in subcorneal, intraepidermal, or follicular locations to form pustules. Small pustules may appear as papules to the naked eye. Intact pustules are often transient in canine skin, probably due to the relative thinness of the canine stratum corneum and epidermis and the frequency of self-trauma. If pustules rupture on the surface, the contents dry, leading to less diagnostic crusted papules.

Collarettes are raised borders of detaching stratum corneum present at the margins of circular areas of inflammation. Although they are evident most commonly as a clinical hallmark of superficial spreading pyoderma, collarettes also can be seen with other less common skin diseases, including pemphigus foliaceus and erythema multiforme.

In deep folliculitis and furunculosis, host response often is more intense, fostering more obvious visible inflammation and swelling that result in **nodule** formation. Nodules usually are erythematous and may hyperpigment with chronicity.

SECONDARY SKIN LESIONS

Pustules either can rupture spontaneously or may be obliterated by self-trauma. Ruptured pustules give rise to **crusted papules**. Because crusted papules can be seen in a wide variety of unrelated skin diseases, their presence is considerably less diagnostic than intact pustules. If multiple crusted papules are grouped, larger areas of crusting composed of dried pus, exudate, and keratin debris may form, resembling generalized crusting or abnormalities of cornification that are seen with a wide variety of other skin diseases.

Self-traumatic **excoriations** secondary to either pruritus or pain are a frequent secondary feature of canine pyoderma. Self-trauma commonly obliterates both the more diagnostic primary lesions of canine pyoderma as well as other secondary lesions such as crusted papules.

Alopecia is an additional frequent sequela to pyoderma. Hair fragments are shed from infected follicles. Presumably, inflammation leads to premature telogenization in infected hair follicles. In addition, transient patchy alopecia affecting nearby noninfected follicles may be caused by localized telogen effluvium and possibly telogen arrest, disrupting the normally asynchronous mosaic hair replacement pattern seen in the dog. Regrowth usually occurs as permanent, scarring alopecia secondary to folliculitis, which is uncommon in the dog, in contrast to the severe scarring seen in humans. Patchy, partial alopecia is clinically noted more frequently in short-coated dogs, but alopecia probably occurs similarly in long-coated dogs but is simply less visible.

> Excellent lighting is essential for a proper physical examination of the skin.

In deep pyoderma, follicular rupture usually leads to more intense inflammation in the surrounding dermis, resulting in larger nodules that can ulcerate and subsequently lead to draining **fistulous tracts.** "Hemorrhagic bullae" are a distinctive clinical feature in some cases of canine deep pyoderma. These lesions result from dermal hemorrhage due to follicular rupture and intense inflammation. Well circumscribed, firm nodules are deep red to dark blue in color. Newer lesions are bright red, signifying fresh hemorrhage. Erosions and ulcers may develop secondary to inflammation, necrosis, and self-traumatic excoriations. Hair loss is seen secondary to follicular inflammation and destruction. Hyperpigmentation and lichenification also are common.

OVERVIEW OF DISTRIBUTION OF LESIONS

Surface pyoderma, where bacterial involvement most likely is purely secondary, exhibits site predilections referable to underlying disease or location of abnormal anatomic skin folds. **Pyotraumatic dermatitis** is seen most commonly in the dorsal lumbosacral region and the lateral thighs. This distribution pattern is assumed to directly correlate with these locations being major sites of the predominant underlying disease, flea allergy dermatitis. Lesions may also occur near the ears or anal sacs in cases not initiated by flea allergy dermatitis. **Intertrigo** or **skin-fold pyoderma** is seen at the specific site of the anatomic defect in a predisposed breed. **Mucocutaneous pyoderma** occurs predominantly on and around the lips but also may affect other mucocutaneous junctions. The cause of mucocutaneous pyoderma and the reasons leading to this distribution pattern are not known.

Uncomplicated primary canine superficial pyoderma occurs most commonly in the moist intertriginous zones of the groin, axilla, and interdigital webs. Frictional microtrauma, moisture accumulation, and heat retention may be predisposing factors. Obesity, if present, is a further contributing cause. **Impetigo** consists of rather mildly inflamed nonfollicular pustules located primarily in the groin and axilla of prepubescent dogs.

In **superficial folliculitis,** crusted papules and pustules are present in greatest density in the intertriginous zones such as the groin and axilla. Inflammation, alopecia, crusting, and pruritus are all variable, influencing both the character and distribution of lesions. Superficial folliculitis may be more generalized on the thorax. The attendant patchy, partial alopecia is more distinctive in short-coated dogs. Improper usage of corticosteroids or other causes of immunosuppression may contribute to the more generalized truncal spread of folliculitis while paradoxically decreasing visible inflammation.

Deep folliculitis and **furunculosis** commonly develops as an extension of superficial folliculitis. Consequently, the distribution pattern may mirror superficial folliculitis but extend further as the disease progresses. Deep pyoderma secondary to demodicosis mimics the distribution pattern of the underlying disease and often severely affects the distal extremities.

Special characteristic distribution patterns aid in the diagnosis of some deep pyodermas. For example, a subgroup recently termed **pyotraumatic folliculitis** seen on the face and elsewhere in certain densely coated large-breed dogs closely mimics pyotraumatic dermatitis clinically. The lesions of **canine acne** develop on the chin in young, short-coated breeds, and **callus pyoderma** develops in calluses over bony prominences or pressure points.

SUGGESTED READINGS

Gross TL, Ihrke PJ, Walder EJ: *Veterinary Dermatopathology: A Macroscopic and Microscopic Evaluation of Canine and Feline Skin Disease.* St. Louis, Mosby–Year Book, 1992, pp 10–14, 238–240, 252–255.

Ihrke PJ: An overview of bacterial skin disease in the dog. Br Vet J 433:112–118, 1987.

Mason I: Pustules and crusted papules, in Locke PH, Harvey RG, Mason IS (eds): *Manual of Small Animal Dermatology.* Gloucestershire, BSAVA, 1993, pp 60–64.

Scott DW, Miller WH, Griffin CE: *Muller & Kirk's Small Animal Dermatology,* ed 5. Philadelphia, WB Saunders, 1995, pp 279–328.

> Improper usage of corticosteroids or other causes of immunosuppression may contribute to the more generalized truncal spread of folliculitis while paradoxically decreasing visible inflammation.

Chapter 6

Surface Pyoderma

PYOTRAUMATIC DERMATITIS
General Considerations

Pyotraumatic dermatitis (acute moist dermatitis, hot spots) is a common, self-induced traumatic canine skin disease with secondary bacterial involvement. Presumably, a vicious itch–scratch cycle is initiated by the underlying pruritus, which usually is induced by allergy, especially flea allergy dermatitis. Other allergic skin diseases, other ectoparasitic diseases, otitis externa, and anal sacculitis occasionally have been implicated as causes of pyotraumatic dermatitis in dogs. A marked seasonality is recognized, with most cases occurring in warm, humid weather. The lesions are quite characteristic clinically and appear to be caused by a combination of focally directed intense self-trauma and secondary surface bacterial suppuration.[1,2] Although strikingly similar visually, pyotraumatic dermatitis is distinct from pyotraumatic folliculitis, a painful or pruritic, usually multicentric deep pyoderma. This syndrome is characterized by a superimposed, self-traumatic pyotraumatic dermatitis–like lesion that is created overlying deep infection[1-3] (see Chapter 8).

Clinical Findings

Pyotraumatic dermatitis develops rapidly. Sharply demarcated erythematous, slightly elevated plaques form in response to severe self-trauma (Figure 6-1). The cause of the strikingly well-demarcated margins is not known. Hair on the lesion is removed by the concerted self-trauma, which leads to secondary erosions and ulcerations. Adherent, viscid debris mats the surrounding hair. Multiple lesions may occur, but satellite lesions are rare. Pain or pruritus is a consistent feature. Most lesions are located at the site of an underlying pruritic or painful process. Consequently, most lesions are located on the caudal lumbosacral region—the most commonly affected site in cases of severe canine flea allergy dermatitis.

Signalment Predilections

The German shepherd, golden retriever, Labrador retriever, collie, Saint Bernard, and other large, densely coated breeds with a heavy undercoat are at increased risk for developing the disease.[1,2] Age or sex predilections have not been noted.

Differential Diagnosis and Diagnosis

Clinical diagnostic differentials include pyotraumatic folliculitis, demodicosis, and neoplasia (especially sweat gland adenocarcinoma and cutaneous metastasis). In addition, fixed drug eruption, an early necrotizing form of idiopathic nodular panniculitis, early localized vasculitis, focal *Malassezia* dermatitis, and candidiasis may appear somewhat visually similar early in the course of disease but are less common.

Diagnosis is usually not difficult and is confirmed by response to therapy. The characteristic clinical features that occur rapidly in a breed at risk with a history of severe self-trauma usually establish the diagnosis. A smear of the exudate stained with a rapid stain should confirm mixed bacterial (predominantly cocci) colonization with degenerating neutrophils. The presence of satellite lesions indi-

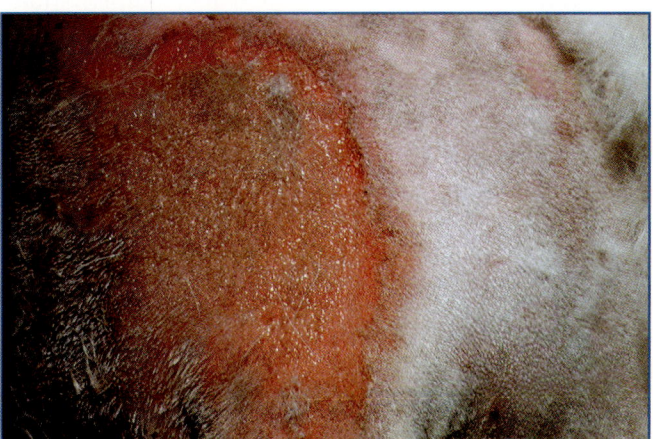

FIGURE 6-1 *Pyotraumatic dermatitis in an adult Samoyed with flea allergy dermatitis. Note the well-demarcated region of erythema and exudation. (Courtesy of Drs. Alan Mundell and Helen Power, case material, University of California.)*

cates the need for further diagnostic evaluation and may signify an alternative primary eruptive process. Skin biopsy should be considered in dogs with unusual clinical features and in dogs unresponsive to palliative therapy based on presumptive diagnosis.

Histopathologic findings include severe erosion and ulceration with exudation. Superficial crusts contain necrotic epidermal debris, degenerating neutrophils, and serum. The adherent crusts may be intensely colonized by gram-positive staphylococci. Lesions are usually sharply demarcated. Moderate neutrophilic inflammation and edema are present and underlie erosion and ulceration.[1]

Therapeutic Overview and Prognosis

Identification and correction of predisposing factors are paramount in achieving successful clinical resolution and preventing recurrence. Because individual lesions respond readily to palliative therapy, prognosis is good if predisposing factors can be determined and corrected. However, recurrence is common if underlying diseases either are not identified or are not managed effectively. In locales where fleas are common, flea allergy dermatitis should be considered the most likely underlying disease until proven otherwise, especially if the lesions occur in the dorsocaudal region.

Lesions should be gently clipped and cleansed. Tranquilization or anesthesia may be required if lesions are severe. A hypoallergenic shampoo[a,b] or gentle antibacterial shampoo containing chlorhexidine[c] or ethyl lactate[d] should be used to remove all debris and exudation from lesions. Topical nonocclusive products containing a drying agent or astringent with or without a corticosteroid should be used daily for 7 to 10 days. Systemic corticosteroids (prednisolone or prednisone, 0.5–1.1 mg/kg/day for 5–7 days) are indicated as adjunctive antiinflammatory therapy in most cases.

INTERTRIGO
General Considerations

Intertrigo or **skin-fold pyoderma** develops as a result of anatomic defects that create a moist, warm environment, which allows intense surface bacterial colonization to occur. The term *intertrigo* is preferred because this syndrome is not a true pyoderma.[2] Lesions develop where folds of skin (usually near mucocutaneous junctions that contribute moisture) retain excretions and secretions, allowing for secondary bacterial overgrowth. Friction between the apposing folds is an additional crucial feature. Erosion and ulceration follow maceration. Lip-fold, facial-fold, vulvar-fold, and tail-fold intertrigo are localized. More generalized-fold dermatitis may be seen in the Chinese shar-pei, with excess dermal mucin contributing to deep, boggy folds. Similar lesions may be seen in folds that are formed secondary to obesity. *Malassezia* organisms can also be found in the surface debris in some dogs with intertrigo and probably also contribute to the inflammatory process.

Clinical Findings

Erythema and slight exudation are the earliest clinical signs of intertrigo. Lesions gradually extend to envelop the affected fold, and exudation increases with chronicity. Erosions and ulcers can be seen in more severely affected dogs. A drainage-board effect may be seen, especially with facial-fold intertrigo, where nonfolded skin below the fold can be erythematous and exudative. Intertrigo may be markedly odoriferous. Secondary hyperpigmentation may occur in breeds predisposed to postinflammatory hyperpigmentation. Pruritus is a common feature of all subgroups of intertrigo. Partially bilaterally symmetric lesions usually are seen with lip-fold and facial-fold intertrigo.

Additional clinical signs can be seen and are contingent on the site of the skin fold. For example, dogs with lip-fold intertrigo are often presented with a tentative diagnosis of severe halitosis, since fold lesions may be minimal and go unnoticed. Owners may resist accepting that such an extreme odor emanates from small folds of skin. Corneal ulceration may be seen secondary to facial-fold intertrigo, since affected dogs scratch and rub the folds of skin between the nose and eyes. Pain may supersede pruritus in cases of vulvar-fold and tail-fold intertrigo. According to Scott and others, "ascending bacterial urinary tract infections are a common sequela to vulvar-fold

> In pyotraumatic dermatitis, a smear of the exudate stained with a rapid stain should confirm mixed bacterial (predominantly cocci) colonization with degenerating neutrophils.

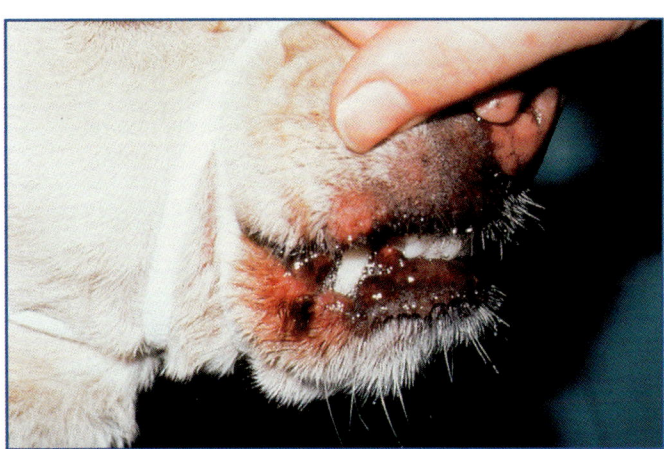

FIGURE 6-2 Lip-fold intertrigo in a crossbreed dog. Odor associated with maceration and secondary bacterial overgrowth in the lip fold were the primary reasons for referral.

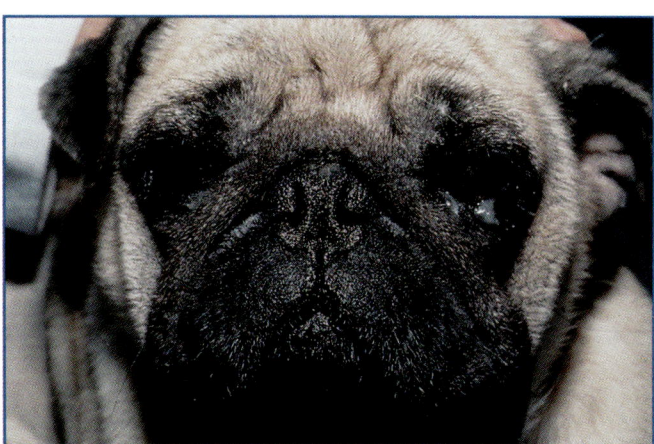

FIGURE 6-3 Facial-fold intertrigo in a pug. The lesions are not visible unless the folds are spread (see Figure 6-4). Facial pruritus was the presenting complaint. (Courtesy of Dr. Alan Mundell, case material, University of California.)

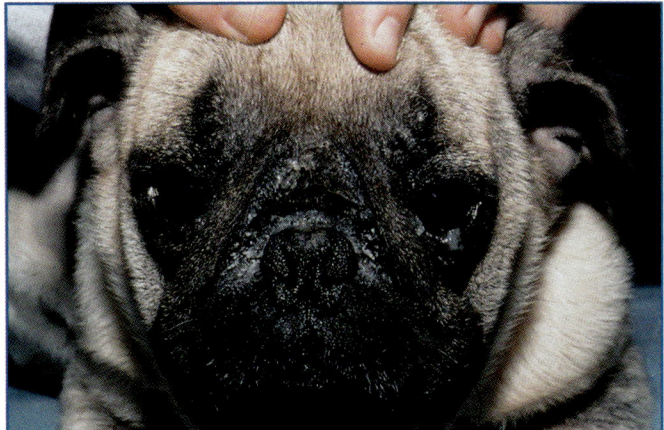

FIGURE 6-4 Facial-fold intertrigo in the pug shown in Figure 6-3. Exposure of the fold reveals maceration and exudation. (Courtesy of Dr. Alan Mundell, case material, University of California.)

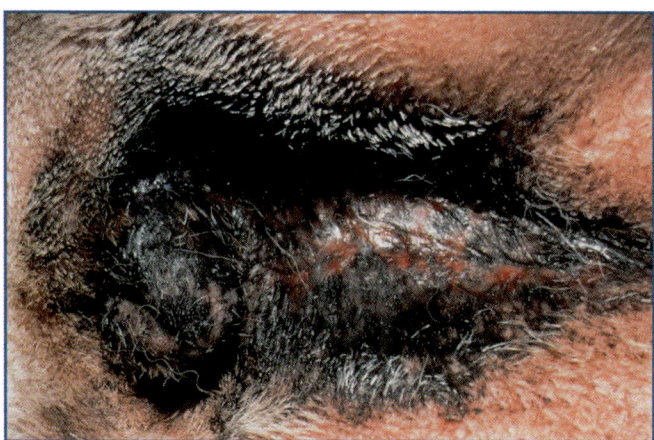

FIGURE 6-5 Severe perivulvar-fold intertrigo in a 10-year-old German shepherd. Note the lichenification and hyperpigmentation, which are hallmarks of chronicity. (Courtesy of Dr. Thierry Olivry, case material, University of California.)

intertrigo."[2] Dogs with tail-fold intertrigo may be presented for intractable perianal self-trauma.

Severity of involvement varies widely from dog to dog. The depth, surface area, and "tightness" of the fold are intrinsic variables that affect the severity of the intertrigo. In addition, in bristle-haired short-coated dogs such as the Chinese shar-pei, friction and irritation caused by hairs rubbing against apposing surfaces may greatly exacerbate intertrigo. External exacerbating factors include increased temperature and humidity.

Signalment Predilections

Striking breed predilections correlate with the specific sites of intertrigo. Lip-fold intertrigo is seen predominantly in springer spaniels, cocker spaniels, Saint Bernards, and Irish setters (Figure 6-2). These breeds share the predisposing anatomic abnormality of a deep, dependent lip fold. Facial-fold intertrigo is seen predominantly in brachycephalic dogs (Figures 6-3 and 6-4). Vulvar-fold intertrigo is believed to occur predominantly in obese bitches with juvenile vulvar conformation that have been spayed before their first heat cycle (Figure 6-5). Tail-fold intertrigo is seen in breeds with corkscrew tails, such as the English bulldog and Boston terrier, with a deep crypt surrounding the base of the tail (Figures 6-6 and 6-7). Generalized intertrigo occurs most commonly in the Chinese shar-pei (Figure 6-8). Similar lesions have been seen in conjunction with obesity in basset hounds and in a variety of other breeds, including the beagle and dachshund. Age predilections have not been reported, but

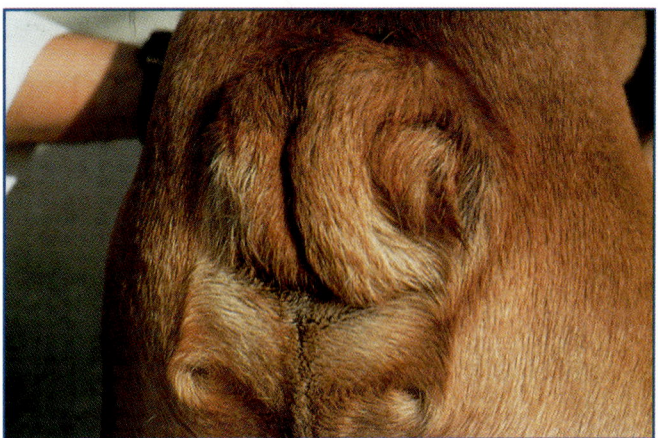

FIGURE 6-6 *Tail-fold intertrigo in a corkscrew-tailed dog. Note that lesions are not visible when the tail is carried in the natural position.*

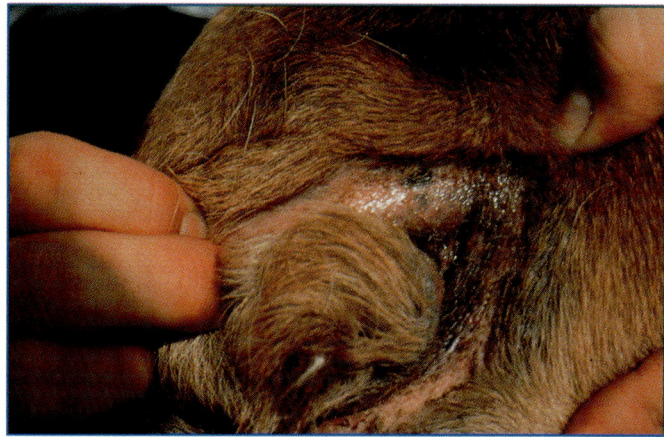

FIGURE 6-7 *Closer view of the dog seen in Figure 6-6, with the tail retracted to show the intertrigo.*

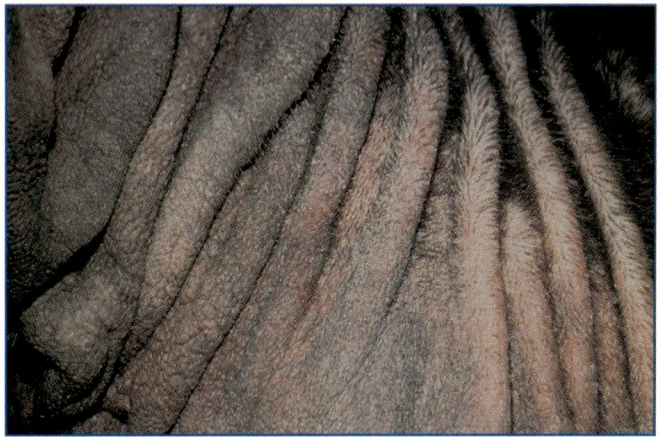

FIGURE 6-8 *Chinese shar-pei with generalized intertrigo seen in conjunction with excess dermal mucin in this breed. (Courtesy of Dr. Lynn Schmeitzel, case material, University of California.)*

untreated intertrigo may increase in severity with time as chronic changes occur.

Differential Diagnosis and Diagnosis

Diagnosis of intertrigo usually is not difficult. Marked breed predilections and compatible history and clinical findings establish a tentative diagnosis because few other diseases localize almost entirely to a skin fold. However, *Malassezia* dermatitis may mimic or coexist with bacterial intertrigo. Consequently, an impression smear for bacteria and *Malassezia* always is recommended. In addition, skin scrapings should always be performed on dogs with lip-fold and facial-fold intertrigo to rule out localized demodicosis. Beyond these minimal diagnostic procedures, most cases of intertrigo are treated based on clinical impression.

Further diagnostic procedures, such as skin biopsy, are performed only if dogs do not respond to appropriate therapy. Skin biopsy is used primarily to rule out other diseases. Intertrigo is characterized histologically by a hyperplastic epidermis with variable superficial pustulation and crusting. Erosion or ulceration may be present. Mild to moderate superficial dermal inflammation is an admixture of plasma cells, lymphocytes, neutrophils, and macrophages.

Diagnostic differentials other than *Malassezia* dermatitis and demodicosis are contingent on the specific anatomic site. Lip-fold intertrigo can be mimicked by localized demodicosis, superficial necrolytic dermatitis (with or without *Malassezia* dermatitis or candidiasis), zinc-responsive dermatosis (especially in the Siberian husky and Alaskan malamute), and early muzzle folliculitis and furunculosis (canine acne). Fixed drug eruption, localized pemphigus foliaceus, early pemphigus vulgaris, and early bullous pemphigoid have been known to be localized to or originate in the lip-fold but rarely occur.

Localized demodicosis, *Malassezia* dermatitis, and dermatophytosis can mimic facial-fold intertrigo. Lesions that are visually similar to vulvar-fold intertrigo have been noted with urinary tract infection with secondary self-trauma, ulcerative dermatosis of the Shetland sheepdog and collie, drug eruptions, canine familial dermatomyositis, and early pemphigus vulgaris and bullous pemphigoid. Tail-fold irritation secondary to flea allergy dermatitis may appear similar to or aggravate tail-fold intertrigo.

Therapeutic Overview and Prognosis

Treatment of skin-fold intertrigo is predominantly palliative unless owners agree to surgical ablation of the anatomic defect initiating the problem. However, because

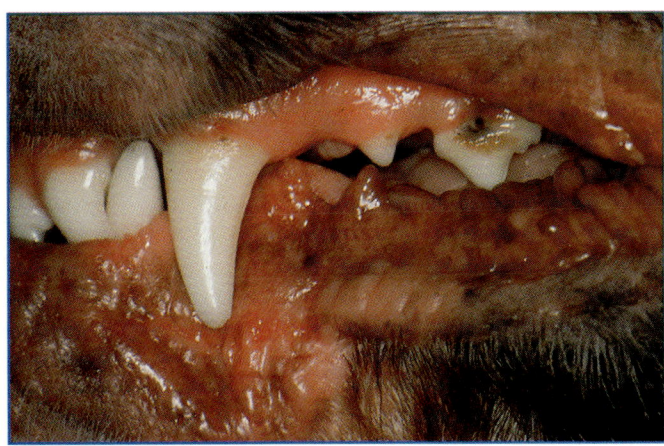

FIGURE 6-9 *Mucocutaneous pyoderma in a crossbreed dog. Note that the lesions involve the lips as well as the lip fold.*

of the availability of newer topical formulations, long-term medical management of intertrigo frequently is more successful today than in the past. Conservative topical medical management (which is essential before surgery can be performed) is always recommended initially, regardless of whether surgery is considered.

Cheiloplasty is curative for lip-fold intertrigo but usually is recommended only for severe cases because medical management routinely is successful. Facial-fold intertrigo typically is managed medically because curative surgery can markedly alter breed recognition. Vulvoplasty (episioplasty) is recommended in dogs with vulvar-fold pyoderma that do not respond to a combination of medical management and weight reduction. Dogs with tail-fold intertrigo affecting a deep, tight crypt generally do not respond to conservative medical management and require complicated surgery that combines fold ablation and tail amputation. Referral to a surgeon for this procedure is recommended.

Medical management initially requires an assessment of the severity of the fold problem. Clipping the hair from the affected area is recommended in long-coated dogs. Clipping may be problematic in short-coated dogs because clipped hairs may create more friction and inflammation in the fold. The affected area is gently cleansed with an antibacterial shampoo that contains benzoyl peroxide and sulfur,[e] benzoyl peroxide,[f-h] chlorhexidine,[c,i] or ethyl lactate.[j] Initially, the affected area is cleansed daily. After several weeks, use can be diminished to twice weekly and finally weekly on a maintenance basis. A topical antibiotic preparation containing mupirocin[k] can be applied sparingly to the fold after cleansing.

MUCOCUTANEOUS PYODERMA
General Considerations

Mucocutaneous pyoderma is an uncommon to rare syndrome characterized clinically by swelling around mucocutaneous junctions with erythema and adherent crusting.[1,4] Certain clinical and histologic features are similar to those found in intertrigo, but lesions are not confined to skin folds and do not originate in folded skin. The syndrome usually affects the lips and perioral skin but occasionally affects other mucocutaneous junctions. Predisposing factors are not known, although response to antibacterial therapy supports a bacterial role in the etiology of the disorder. Relapses are common. Mucocutaneous pyoderma of the lips and perioral skin is clinically distinct from lip-fold intertrigo but may coexist with lip-fold intertrigo.

Clinical Findings

Mucocutaneous pyoderma is gradual in onset. Erythema and swelling precede crusting as the initial clinical signs. Crusts entrap hairs at affected mucocutaneous junctions. Affected lips are markedly erythematous and uniformly swollen (Figure 6-9). The lateral commissures frequently are affected. Fissuring and erosions with adherent crusting are present in more severe cases. Lip and perioral lesions commonly are bilaterally symmetric. Salivary staining may surround the lip lesions, and tenacious exudate may mat the surrounding hair. Depigmentation of the lips is noted in chronic cases. The mucocutaneous junction of one or both nares of the planum nasale may be affected. Bilateral symmetry is not seen in lesions involving the nares. Pruritus is mild to moderate, and pain may be present. Affected dogs may rub their faces on carpeting or furniture. Dogs with more severe lesions resent palpation and examination. Mild odor

> Mucocutaneous pyoderma is an uncommon to rare syndrome characterized clinically by swelling around mucocutaneous junctions with erythema and adherent crusting.

may be associated with the lesions, but, overall, odor is not as striking a feature as with lip-fold intertrigo. Regional lymphadenopathy may be present. Similar lesions can affect the vulva, prepuce, or anus but are less common.

Signalment Predilections

German shepherds may be at increased risk for mucocutaneous pyoderma. Age or sex predilections have not been noted.

Differential Diagnosis and Diagnosis

Canine mucocutaneous pyoderma affecting the lips and perioral skin is distinctive visually. Lip-fold intertrigo, localized demodicosis, early discoid lupus erythematosus, zinc-responsive dermatosis, generic dog food skin disease, and muzzle folliculitis and furunculosis (canine acne) are possible diagnostic differentials.

Lip-fold pyoderma is confined to the deep triangular folds below each side of the lower lip, whereas mucocutaneous pyoderma commonly involves the entire lips and perioral skin. Localized demodicosis may appear casually similar to mucocutaneous pyoderma, but haired perioral skin rather than the lips is involved. Mucocutaneous pyoderma primarily affecting the lips or the nares may closely mimic early discoid lupus erythematosus. Although lesions may be similar, the swelling of the lips seen with mucocutaneous pyoderma is distinctive and not a clinical feature of canine discoid lupus erythematosus. Early zinc-responsive dermatosis in Alaskan breeds may appear visually similar, but perioral lesions are common.

Skin biopsy may be needed to rule out other diseases. Direct immunofluorescent or immunohistochemical testing may be useful in differentiating mucocutaneous pyoderma from discoid lupus erythematosus.

Mucocutaneous pyoderma is characterized histologically by a hyperplastic epidermis with superficial pustulation and crusting with erosion or ulceration. Lichenoid inflammation with plasma cells, lymphocytes, neutrophils, and macrophages is present in the superficial dermis. Mild inflammation may surround adnexal appendages in the adjacent haired skin.

Therapeutic Overview and Prognosis

Dogs with mild cases of canine mucocutaneous pyoderma respond readily to topical therapy alone, whereas those with more severe cases require combined topical and systemic antibacterial therapy. Long-term clinical management is complicated by frequent recrudescence.

The hair surrounding the lips should be gently clipped to prevent the retention of secretions that mat the surrounding hair. If pain is evident on manipulation in more severe cases, clipping can be delayed until antibacterial shampoos and systemic antibiotics have been utilized and have diminished inflammation. Antibacterial shampoos containing benzoyl peroxide and sulfur[e] or benzoyl peroxide[f-h] are recommended. If irritation is seen with benzoyl peroxide–containing products, a product containing ethyl lactate[j] may be used. The affected area should be gently cleansed once a day for the initial 2 weeks.

A 2% mupirocin ointment[k] is applied sparingly to the lesions after shampooing. This hydrating ointment has been more successful therapeutically than either antibiotic creams or benzoyl peroxide gels. Antibacterial cleansing and the application of topical antibiotics usually can be decreased to twice weekly after 2 weeks of daily therapy. Systemic antibiotics may be administered to more severely affected dogs during the first 3 to 4 weeks of topical therapy.

Therapy may be discontinued in 3 to 4 weeks after all lesions resolve; however, recrudescence is common. Some dogs require long-term maintenance therapy with antibacterial shampoos and mupirocin ointment used on a weekly basis. Systemic antibiotics may be required occasionally in more severe cases.

---

[a]Allergroom®, Allerderm/Virbac.
[b]HyLyte, DVM Pharmaceuticals.
[c]ChlorhexiDerm, DVM Pharmaceuticals.
[d]Etiderm™, Allerderm/Virbac.
[e]Sulf/OxyDex, DVM Pharmaceuticals.
[f]Pyoben®, Allerderm/Virbac.
[g]OxyDex, DVM Pharmaceuticals.
[h]Micro Pearls™ Benzoyl Peroxide Shampoo, Evsco Pharmaceuticals.
[i]Nolvasan®, Fort Dodge.
[j]Etiderm™, Allerderm/Virbac.
[k]Bactoderm®, Pfizer Animal Health.

REFERENCES

1. Gross TL, Ihrke PJ, Walder EJ: *Veterinary Dermatopathology: A Macroscopic and Microscopic Evaluation of Canine and Feline Skin Disease.* St. Louis, Mosby–Year Book, 1992, pp 58–59, 141–143.
2. Scott DW, Miller WH, Griffin CE: *Muller & Kirk's Small Animal Dermatology,* ed 5. Philadelphia, WB Saunders, 1995, pp 883–887.
3. Reinke SI, Stannard AA, Ihrke PJ, et al: Histopathologic features of pyotraumatic dermatitis. JAVMA 190:57–60, 1987.
4. Ihrke PJ, Gross TL: Canine mucocutaneous pyoderma, in Bonagura JD (ed): *Kirk's Current Veterinary Therapy XII.* Philadelphia, WB Saunders, 1995, pp 618–619.

Chapter 7

Superficial Pyoderma

IMPETIGO

General Considerations

Impetigo (puppy pyoderma) is a common, superficial, nonfollicular pustular bacterial skin disease seen predominantly in the glabrous or sparsely haired regions of the groin and axillae in young dogs[1,2] (Figure 7-1). *Staphylococcus intermedius*, as is seen in most canine bacterial skin diseases, is usually the primary pathogen. However, other bacteria such as *Pseudomonas*, *Enterobacter*, and *Escherichia coli* may apparently be the primary pathogens in the bullous form of impetigo seen in conjunction with underlying immunosuppression, usually in older dogs. This phenomenon is evident most frequently with naturally occurring or iatrogenic hyperglucocorticoidism but has also been seen in conjunction with diabetes mellitus, hypothyroidism, lymphoid neoplasia, and other less common debilitating, immunocompromising diseases. Underlying causes usually are not evident in the more common form of impetigo seen in prepubescent and pubescent dogs. Inflammation or enhanced susceptibility secondary to fecal debris, urine scalding, hair coat matting, ectoparasitism, environmental hygiene, or poor nutrition have been suggested to contribute to the disease.[3-9]

> Recovery in young dogs with impetigo usually is hastened by topical therapy and a short course of systemic antibiotics.

Clinical Findings

Crusted papules are the most common lesions seen in cases of canine impetigo because intact pustules are fragile and rupture easily. The pustular contents vary from creamy white to yellow, leading to yellowish crusts that adhere to mildly erythematous papules. Peripheral epidermal collarettes may remain as a "footprint" of pyoderma. The finding of intact, nonfollicular pustules amid widespread crusted papules in the groin or axillae of a young dog is highly suggestive of impetigo (Figures 7-2 and 7-3). A hand lens can aid in determining whether pustules are interfollicular (impetigo) or follicular (folliculitis); follicular pustules will have central protruding hairs. Clinical differentiation is important because dogs with impetigo respond more readily to therapy than those with folliculitis. Partial bilateral symmetry may be seen in the glabrous inguinal and axillary regions.

Pruritus, if present, is mild, and lesions are nonpainful and otherwise asymptomatic. Impetigo may be noted as an incidental finding when young dogs are presented to the veterinarian for other reasons. Many cases of impetigo probably go undiagnosed because owners may be unaware of the skin lesions.

Bullous impetigo is characterized by large, nonfollicular pustules ranging from 5 to 15 mm in diameter (Figure 7-4). Intact pustules usually are flaccid. Content color can vary from white to yellow or even light green. In the author's experience, unusual color in a pustule indicates the likelihood that the responsible organism is something other than *S. intermedius*.

Signalment Predilections

Impetigo is seen predominantly in prepubescent and pubescent dogs. Impetigo in adult or geriatric dogs is uncommon and suggests underlying disease. Breed or sex predilections have not been noted.

Differential Diagnosis and Diagnosis

Diagnostic differentials include predominantly early flea allergy dermatitis and superficial folliculitis. Pruritus should be evident, even with mild flea allergy dermatitis, and the pustules of folliculitis are oriented around hairs and their follicles. A variant of pemphigus foliaceus characterized by intermittent

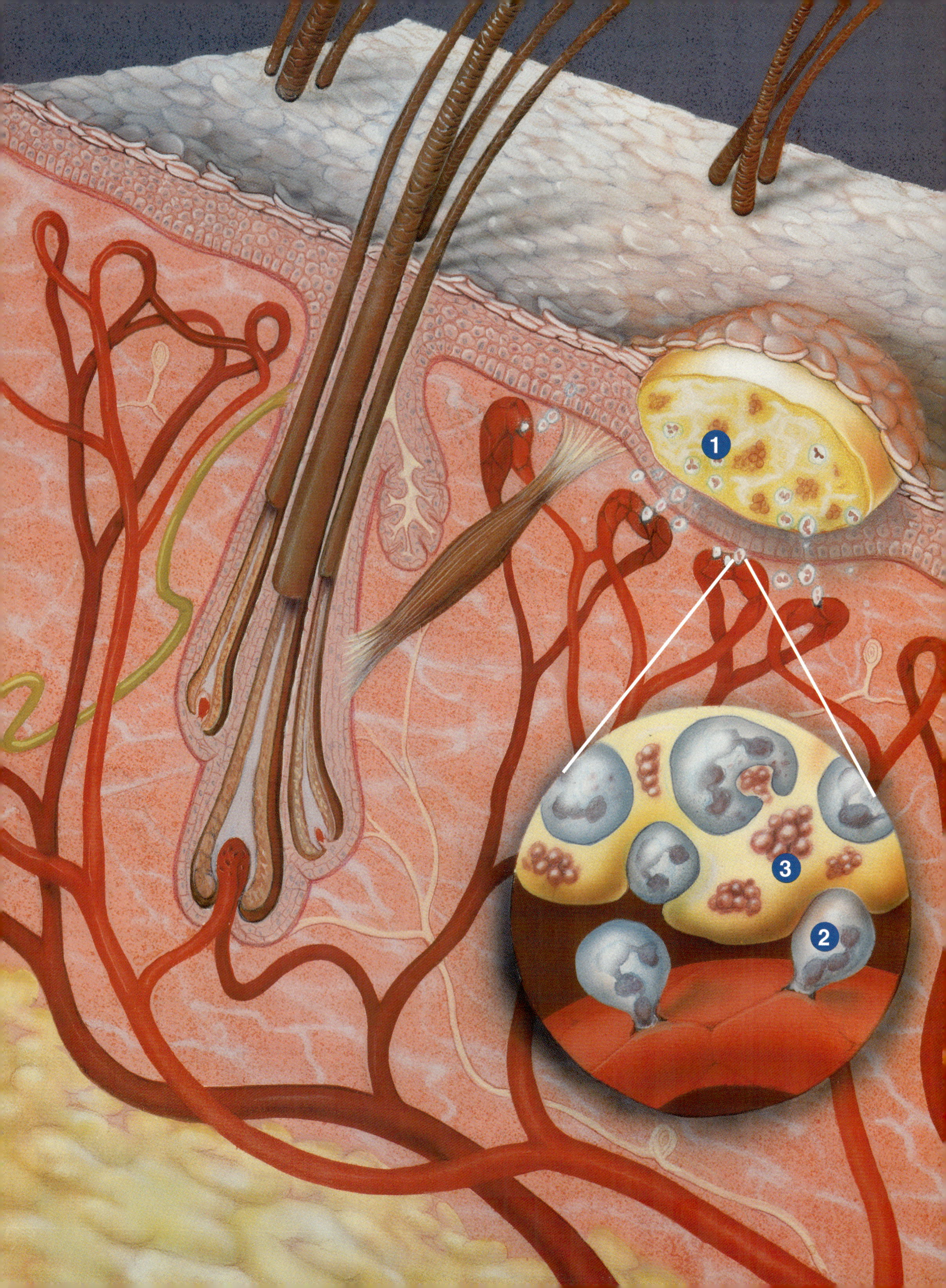
1
2
3

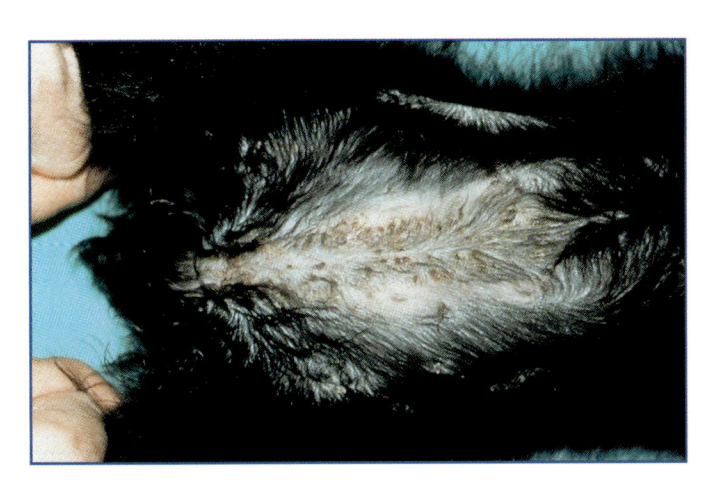

FIGURE 7-2 *Impetigo in a prepubescent dog. Note the generalized distribution of crusted papules and occasional pustules on the ventral abdomen.*

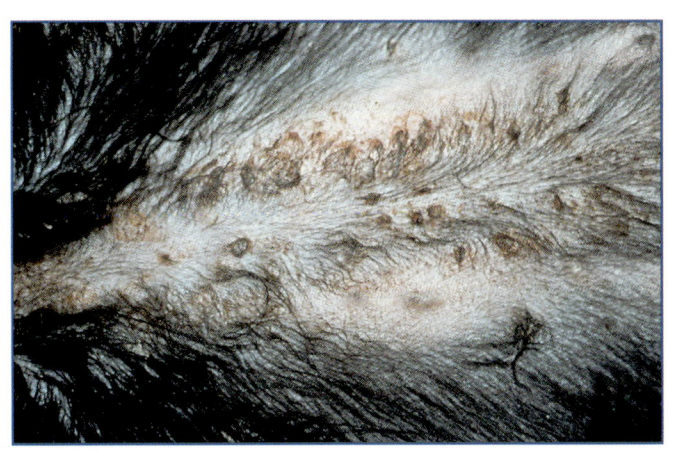

FIGURE 7-3 *Closer view of the dog shown in Figure 7-2. Several intact pustules can be seen among the more common crusted papules that resulted from pustule rupture.*

waves of truncal pustules ranging from 2 to 10 mm in diameter can mimic bullous impetigo.

Diagnosis is not difficult, but clinical impression should be confirmed by smears of the contents of intact pustules. Smears stained with a routine rapid stain should indicate the presence of a moderate to large number of cocci with degenerating neutrophils. The finding of other bacteria warrants bacterial culture, identification, and sensitivity testing. The presence of acantholytic cells, especially in lesions suspected to be bullous impetigo, warrants skin biopsy to rule out the possibility of pemphigus foliaceus. In most circumstances, response to antibacterial therapy definitively establishes the diagnosis.

Skin biopsy should be considered in dogs with unusual clinical features and in dogs unresponsive to appropriate therapy based on presumptive diagnosis. Skin biopsy specimens should be obtained from intact pustules because crusted papules usually represent pustules in advanced stages of degeneration.

Typical histopathologic findings include discrete subcorneal pustules composed predominantly of neutrophils. Pustules usually are elevated above the epidermal surface and are located between hair follicles. In bullous impetigo, pustules may span multiple hair follicles. Special bacterial stains reveal cocci or the initiating organism within intact pustules. The epidermis usually is spongiotic and may be acanthotic. Superficial perivascular to interstitial mixed inflammation is seen in the dermis and is composed predominantly of neutrophils.[7]

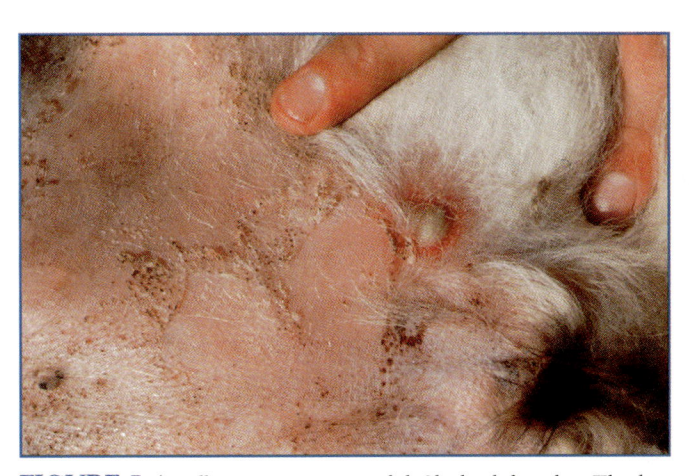

FIGURE 7-4 *Bullous impetigo in an adult Shetland sheepdog. The dog had received frequent doses of injectable corticosteroids for pruritus. Larger-than-usual pustules are seen. The lack of hair emanating from the pustules indicates their nonfollicular origin.*

Therapeutic Overview and Prognosis

Impetigo in young dogs follows a benign, frequently asymptomatic course. Consequently, overly aggressive therapy is not necessary and should be avoided. Spontaneous regression may occur, but recovery in young dogs with impetigo usually is hastened by topical therapy and a short course of systemic antibiotics. Possible contributing factors such as canine hygiene (e.g., fecal debris, urine scalding, and matted hair coat), environmental hygiene, ectoparasitism, or poor nutrition should be addressed, if suspected.

In early cases, or if the lesions are markedly focal and mild, locally applied topical therapy alone may be cura-

---

FIGURE 7-1 *Impetigo. (1) Superficial epidermal nonfollicular pustule, (2) neutrophils migrating intercellularly through the epidermis into the pustule, and (3) staphylococcal bacteria within the pustule.*

tive. Antibacterial shampoos of the affected area and the application of a topical ointment containing mupirocin[a] may be sufficient to cure the disease. The affected area is cleansed gently on a daily basis, and mupirocin is applied sparingly twice daily.

The affected comparatively glabrous groin and axilla of long-coated dogs should be clipped if matting of the hair coat is evident. A gentle antibacterial shampoo containing chlorhexidine[b] or ethyl lactate[c] is recommended. Products containing benzoyl peroxide should be used with caution because they are more likely to cause irritation on the comparatively more tender skin of puppies. Initially, the affected areas should be cleansed daily for the first few days, after which the cleansing should be continued daily or every other day for 10 to 14 days, contingent on the severity of the disease.

Systemic antibiotics usually are not required. However, 10 to 14 days of systemic antibiotic therapy with concurrent topical therapy frequently may speed recovery.

Bullous impetigo in adult or geriatric dogs potentially indicates serious underlying disease. Consequently, testing to evaluate the general and immunologic health of an adult dog with impetigo is recommended. The diagnosis and management of the underlying disease or predisposing cause usually are required for the successful management of bullous impetigo.

Management of bullous impetigo in the adult dog is similar to the management of other types of impetigo, except that systemic antibiotics are always indicated for a minimum of 3 weeks. Benzoyl peroxide–containing shampoos[d-g] may be used as an alternative to shampoos containing ethyl lactate or chlorhexidine.

SUPERFICIAL BACTERIAL FOLLICULITIS
General Considerations

Superficial bacterial folliculitis is the most common canine bacterial skin infection worldwide (Figure 7-5). In regions of the world that do not readily support fleas, superficial bacterial folliculitis is probably the most common canine skin disease.[10,11] *S. intermedius* is the primary pathogen, as is the case in other forms of canine pyoderma. The clinical presentation of superficial folliculitis is highly variable and is probably caused by differences in breed response, individual host resistance, and underlying diseases. As in impetigo, the glabrous skin of the groin and axillae is the most common initial site of involvement. Superficial follicular pustules are the unifying clinical feature.

Frequently, canine bacterial folliculitis is seen secondary to coexistent disease or in conjunction with other predisposing factors. As discussed in Chapter 3, inflammation, obstruction, atrophy, dysplasia, or degeneration of the hair follicles predispose dogs to secondary bacterial folliculitis. Cornification defects (seborrhea) and allergy including atopic dermatitis have been consistently shown to be linked with canine pyoderma (see Chapter 3).[12-17] Other apparently common predisposing diseases or syndromes include hypothyroidism as well as naturally occurring and iatrogenic hyperglucocorticoidism. Other likely predisposing factors include inflammation or pruritus from any source, defects in the immune response, and poor grooming.[2,3] However, the specific initiating factors in the development of pyoderma frequently still are not known (see Chapter 4).

Clinical Findings

The most characteristic clinical feature of canine superficial bacterial folliculitis is an inflammatory pustule centered around the hair follicle (Figures 7-6 and 7-7). Intact pustules arise on erythematous bases and contain white or creamy yellow purulent debris. In dogs with darkly pigmented skin, inflammatory lesions including pustules may be substantially less distinctive. Intact pustules are fragile and rupture easily,

---

FIGURE 7-5 *Superficial folliculitis.* (1) *Follicular pustule localized to the entrance and upper one third of the hair follicle.* (2) *Neutrophils, staphylococcal bacteria, and debris within the follicular pustule.*

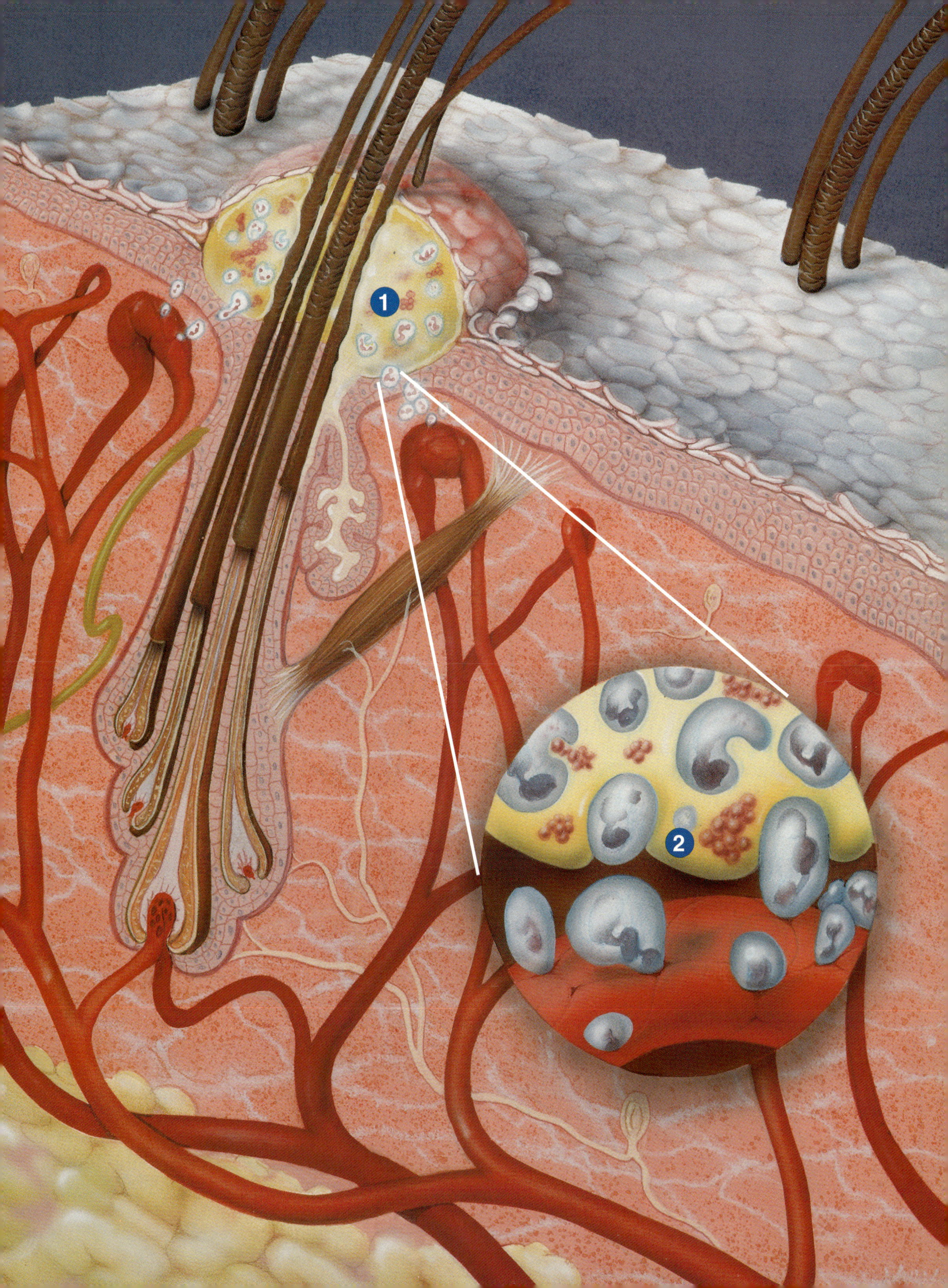
1
2

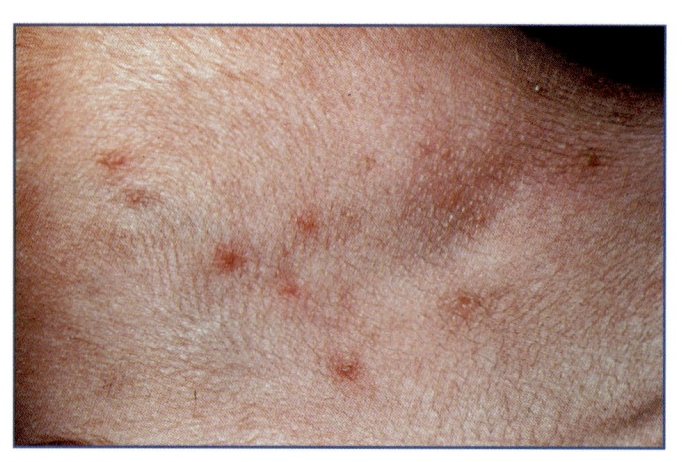

FIGURE 7-6 *Uncomplicated, early superficial folliculitis in the groin of a dachshund. Note both the intact pustules and crusted papules caused by pustule rupture.*

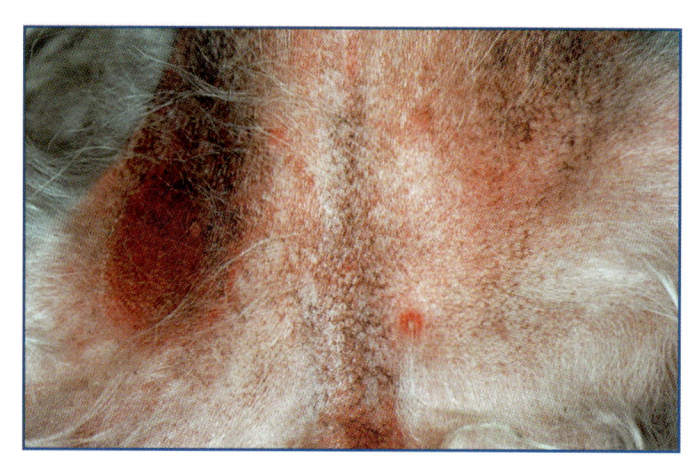

FIGURE 7-7 *Superficial folliculitis in the groin of a dog. Self-trauma induced by pruritus has induced more severe lesions than those seen in Figure 7-6.*

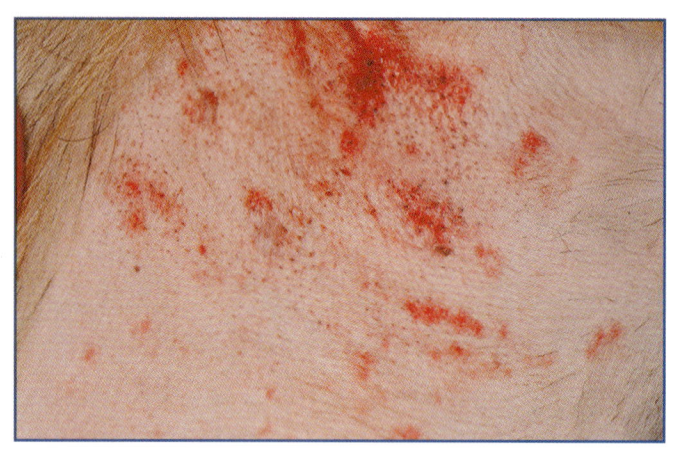

FIGURE 7-8 *Superficial folliculitis secondary to atopic dermatitis and the injudicious use of corticosteroids on the abdomen of a dog.*

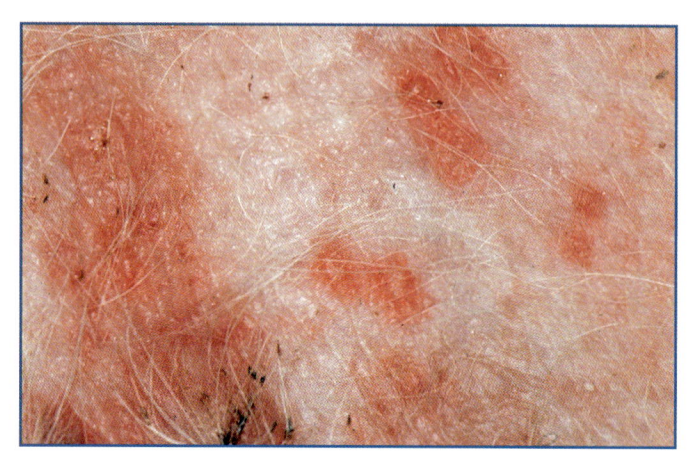

FIGURE 7-9 *Superficial folliculitis located on the comparatively glabrous skin of the ventral abdomen. The follicular orientation of several pustules is indicated by hairs emanating from their center.*

eventually resulting in crusted papules. The papules may not be crusted in appearance because the adherent crust may have been removed by self-trauma or has simply fallen off. Consequently, papules with or without adherent crust, although less diagnostic, may be the most common clinical feature of canine superficial bacterial folliculitis.[3,6,8] Although they are unpredictable clinical features, pruritus and attendant self-trauma are common. Pruritus may or may not correlate with the degree of erythema. Regional lymphadenopathy is a common finding.

The pustules of superficial folliculitis may vary in size but usually are less than 5 mm in diameter, including both the actual encapsulated pus (rarely >2 mm in diameter) and the surrounding raised, erythematous zone. The severity and extent of erythema is quite variable (Figure 7-8). Some pustules may be difficult to identify with the naked eye. A hand lens is useful in determining whether intact pustules have a follicular orientation, as follicular pustules will have central protruding hairs unless the hair has been shed (Figure 7-9). The rupture of pustules may lead to the formation of peripheral collarettes at the pustular margins, which are characterized by a circular peeling back of the superficial keratin layer of the stratum corneum surrounding the site of the ruptured pustule (Figures 7-10 and 7-11). These lesions may indicate superficial spreading pyoderma occurring with superficial bacterial folliculitis.

Hyperpigmentation is markedly variable and tends to follow apparent breed predilections for postinflammatory hyperpigmentation. Hyperpigmented rings may form within the boundaries of the collarette (Figure 7-12). Alternatively, small foci of hyperpigmentation may occur at the follicular ostia, marking the sites of previous folliculitis, and serve as an additional diagnostic aid by indicating the follicular orientation of the inflammation. Postinflamma-

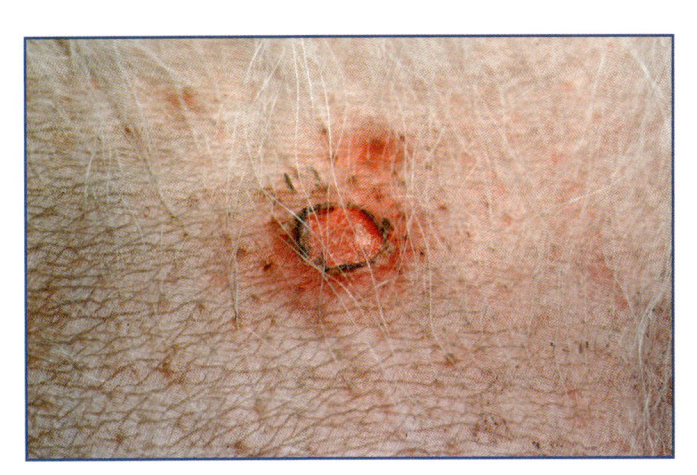

FIGURE 7-10 An epidermal collarette caused by the rupture of a pustule in a dog with superficial folliculitis. Although a number of inflammatory skin diseases can cause peripheral collarettes, pyoderma is the most common cause. (Courtesy of Dr. Ralf Mueller, case material, University of California.)

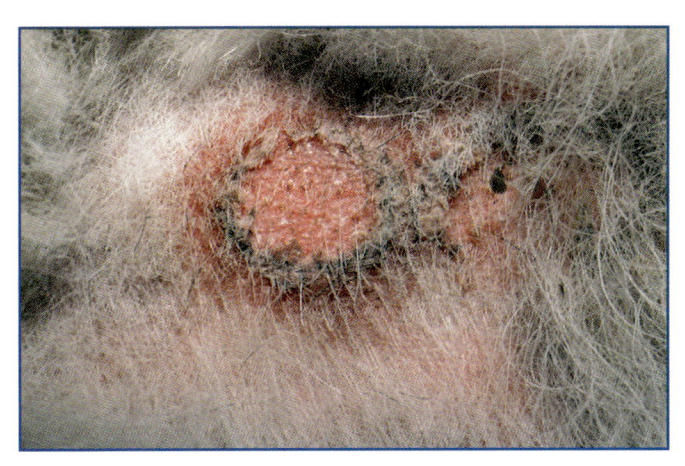

FIGURE 7-11 Coalescing epidermal collarettes in a dog with moderately severe superficial folliculitis. (Courtesy of Dr. Ralf Mueller, case material, University of California.)

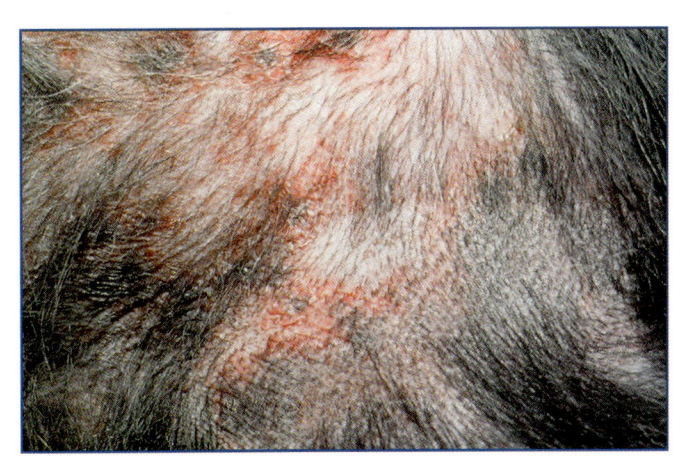

FIGURE 7-12 Superficial folliculitis with epidermal collarettes. Lichenification and hyperpigmentation indicate chronicity. (Courtesy of Dr. Ralf Mueller, case material, University of California.)

tory hyperpigmentation may become confluent with chronicity (Figures 7-13 and 7-14). German shepherds, keeshonds, dachshunds, and brachycephalic breeds such as the mastiff and bullmastiff may become hyperpigmented in response to inflammation more readily than other breeds.

Hair coat abnormalities may precede or coexist with frank hair loss. A disheveled hair coat with small tufts of hair rising above the remainder of the coat may mark the initial stage of folliculitis in a short-coated dog. These elevated hairs presumably are due to inflammation in the vicinity of the erector pili muscles and are suggestive but not diagnostic of focal, mid-dermal inflammation associated with the hair follicle.

Alopecia is a common feature of superficial bacterial folliculitis. Transient, nonscarring alopecia may lead to distinct circular patches of hair loss that form surrounding previously affected hair follicles. Chronicity leads to a generalized "moth-eaten" appearance. This phenomenon is more obvious in short-coated breeds, which has led to use of the term *short-coated dog pyoderma* (Figure 7-15). Focal, postinflammatory hair cycle arrest has been suggested by Stannard as the reason for this transient, distinctive alopecia.[7] Careful examination of the periphery of these patches may reveal individual peripheral collarettes, coalescing collarettes, and crusted papules more indicative of bacterial infection. Hair loss appears more gradual and clinically subtle in long-coated dogs and may not be noted by the owner until a generalized thinning and dishevelment of the affected area leads to closer examination.[9]

Larger, more firm, crusted papules, pustules, or nodules mimicking deep pyoderma may be seen occasionally in dogs with superficial bacterial folliculitis. These firm, well-demarcated lesions may indicate the less common histologic changes seen in dogs with superficial perforating folliculitis.[7]

The comparatively glabrous inguinal and axillary regions are the most common initial sites for the development of canine superficial bacterial folliculitis. Both the dorsal and ventral interdigital webs are additional predisposed sites in some breeds. Superficial bacterial folliculitis may generalize. This phenomenon occurs commonly in dogs with iatrogenic or naturally occurring hyperglucocorticoidism but may be seen with other conditions characterized by diminished immunologic surveillance.

Signalment Predilections

Superficial bacterial folliculitis may be seen in any breed. If infection is secondary to predisposing disease,

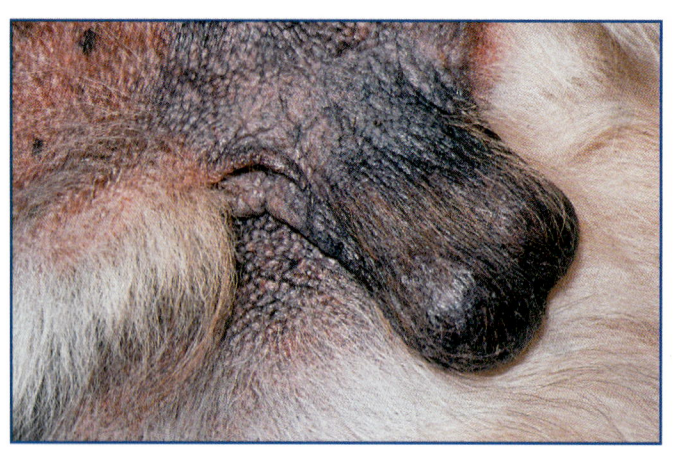

FIGURE 7-13 Chronic superficial folliculitis predominantly affecting the groin of a German shepherd. Exudation, lichenification, and extensive hyperpigmentation are present.

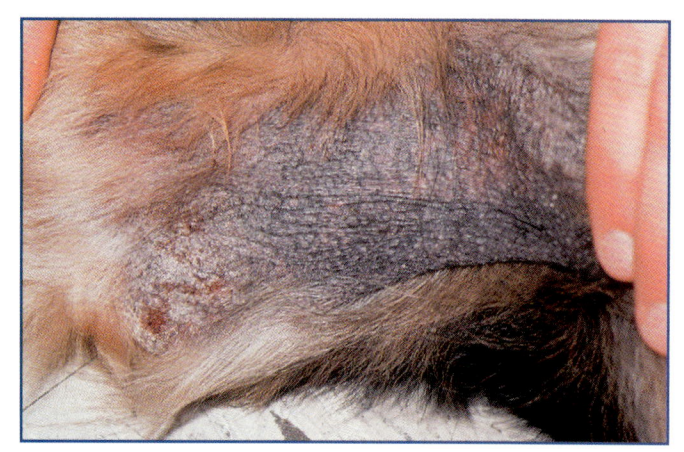

FIGURE 7-14 Closer view of the lesions seen in Figure 7-13. Superficial pyoderma may be difficult to diagnose in dogs with extensive chronic lesions.

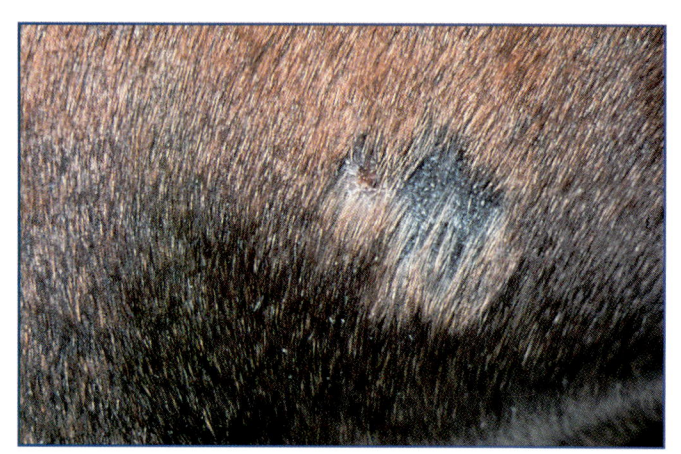

FIGURE 7-15 Superficial bacterial folliculitis in a short-coated dog (dachshund). Note the circular patch of alopecia.

breed predilections may parallel those of the predisposing disease. Age or sex predilections have not been noted.

Differential Diagnosis and Diagnosis

Diagnostic differentials vary with clinical presentation. Since much canine superficial bacterial folliculitis is secondary to underlying causes, long-term therapeutic success frequently requires both the diagnosis and management of underlying problems.

If intact follicular pustules are present, bacterial folliculitis is the most likely diagnosis because pyoderma is by far the most common cause of canine folliculitis. Other causes of canine follicular pustular disease include demodicosis and, much less commonly, dermatophytosis. The vesicopustules seen with canine pemphigus foliaceus may span hair follicles, also mimicking folliculitis. Impetigo can mimic bacterial folliculitis if the presence or absence of follicular orientation is not easily determined on glabrous skin. The rare pustular disease, sterile eosinophilic pustulosis, and the controversial disease, subcorneal pustular dermatosis, can also mimic bacterial folliculitis.

If only papules and crusted papules are present, diagnostic differentials include impetigo, flea allergy dermatitis, demodicosis, sarcoptic acariasis, and numerous other less common diseases characterized by a papular rash. Peripheral epidermal collarettes suggestive of superficial bacterial folliculitis also can be seen with superficial spreading pyoderma, impetigo, pemphigus foliaceus, and erythema multiforme. The possibility of superficial spreading pyoderma coexisting with superficial folliculitis should be considered if the pustules are accompanied by prominent collarette formation without previous central pustule formation.

Superficial bacterial folliculitis must be differentiated from urticaria in short-coated dogs if tufting of a small group of hairs above the surrounding hair coat is noted. Both pathologic processes can cause elevated tufts of hairs and patchy, partial alopecia. Urticaria should be more rapid in onset and more transient, but differentiation may be challenging if frank pustules or suspicious crusted papules are not observed.

Diagnosis is accomplished by the microscopic examination of smears from pustules, skin scrapings, dermatophyte culture, bacterial culture, histopathology, and, frequently, response to therapy. The minimum data base required to establish the diagnosis of superficial folliculitis varies due to the pleomorphic clinical presentation.

If intact pustules are present, smears of pustular contents should be stained with a rapid stain and evaluated for the presence of a moderate to large number of cocci and activated neutrophils. The finding of other bacteria warrants bacterial culture, identification, and sensitivity testing. The presence of acantholytic cells in smears from apparent pustules necessitates skin biopsy to rule out pemphigus foliaceus.

Skin scrapings should always be performed to rule out demodicosis. Since dermatophytosis may resemble bacterial folliculitis, microscopic hair examination and dermatophyte cultures also may be beneficial.

If unusual clinical features are present or a dog has not responded to appropriate therapy based on a presumptive diagnosis of pyoderma, skin biopsy should be performed. Ideally, skin biopsy specimens should be obtained from recently formed, intact pustules, since crusted papules frequently yield less diagnostic information.

Common histopathologic features of superficial bacterial folliculitis include the formation of pustules within the infundibulum or ostium of hair follicles with neutrophilic and occasionally eosinophilic inflammation. Mild exocytosis may be present. Dermal inflammation and edema are variable. Some free keratin indicative of occasional follicular rupture may be present. Chronic lesions are characterized by perifollicular and perivascular infiltration of plasma cells, macrophages, and a lesser number of neutrophils. Perifollicular fibrosis may be present in more severe lesions. Both affected and surrounding hair follicles frequently are in telogen phase, possibly due to telogen arrest.[7]

Therapeutic Overview and Prognosis

Superficial bacterial folliculitis is a highly variable disease. Since canine bacterial folliculitis often occurs secondary to coexistent disease or other predisposing factors, recrudescence is likely if these factors either are not identified or cannot be managed effectively. Consequently, required therapy and prognosis vary widely from case to case. Systemic antibiotic therapy is almost always necessary to achieve therapeutic success. Three weeks of appropriate systemic antibiotic therapy usually is sufficient to achieve clinical remission in immunologically competent dogs (see Chapter 10).

> Chronic lesions of superficial bacterial folliculitis are characterized by perifollicular and perivascular infiltration of plasma cells, macrophages, and a lesser number of neutrophils.

Adjunctive topical therapy, although not required, is beneficial and may enhance speed of recovery, diminish the likelihood of recurrence, and improve patient attitude.[18,19] Potentially beneficial antibacterial shampoos include those containing benzoyl peroxide and sulfur,[d] benzoyl peroxide,[e-g] ethyl lactate,[c] and chlorhexidine.[b] Ideally, the entire dog should be bathed. Frequency of shampoo varies with the severity of the infection, but, in general, the dog should be bathed either once or twice a week.

Occasionally, superficial bacterial folliculitis may be mild and very localized. In these cases, locally applied topical therapy may be sufficient. Antibacterial shampoos of the affected area and the application of a topical ointment containing mupirocin[a] may be sufficient for cure. The localized, affected area is cleansed gently on a daily basis with an antibacterial shampoo, and mupirocin is applied sparingly twice daily.

SUPERFICIAL SPREADING PYODERMA
General Considerations

Superficial spreading pyoderma is a common canine superficial bacterial skin disease (Figure 7-16). *S. intermedius* is the primary pathogen as is the case in other types of canine pyoderma. This syndrome may be seen either alone or in conjunction with superficial bacterial folliculitis. The frequent localization of lesions to the glabrous intertriginous regions of the groin and axillae suggests that moisture and heat retention and frictional microtrauma may predispose dogs to the development of superficial spreading pyoderma.[7,20] Superficial spreading pyoderma may be seen secondary to underlying diseases or other predisposing factors similar to those in dogs with superficial folliculitis. Underlying allergic disease may be the major predisposition.

Clinical Findings

Multiple erythematous macules enlarge centripetally from point sources and create expanding erythematous rings with well-demarcated, peeling, scaling borders (Figures 7-17 to 7-19). The macules commonly achieve diameters of 1 to 2.5 cm. Distinctive epidermal collarettes form

1
2
3

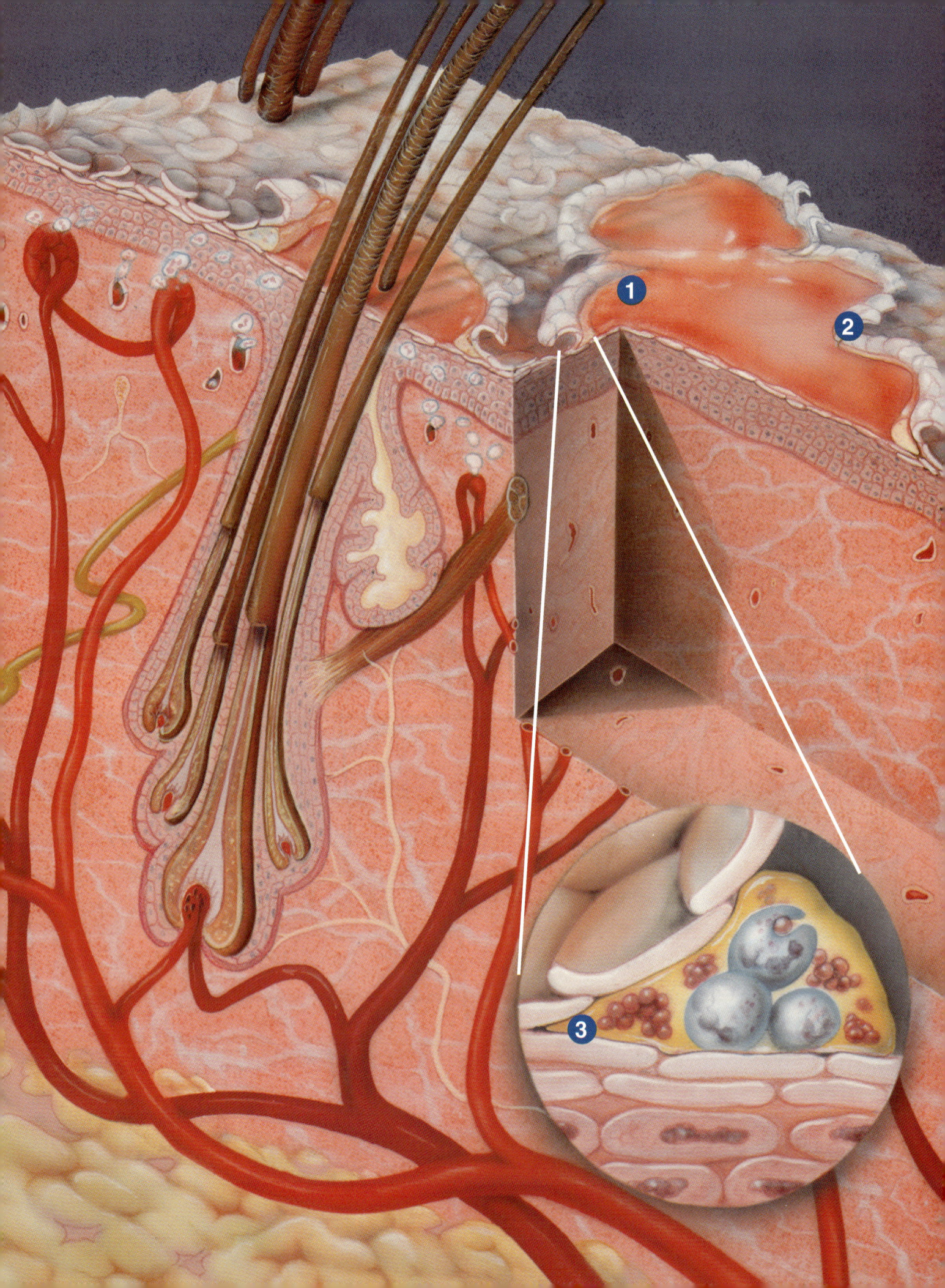

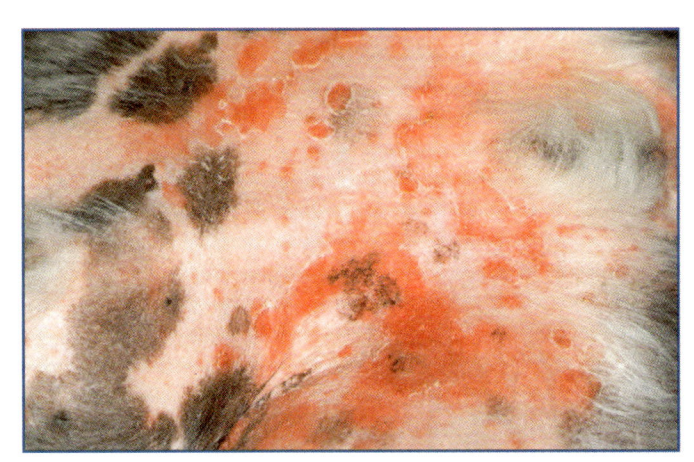

FIGURE 7-17 *Superficial spreading pyoderma on the abdomen of a Border collie.*

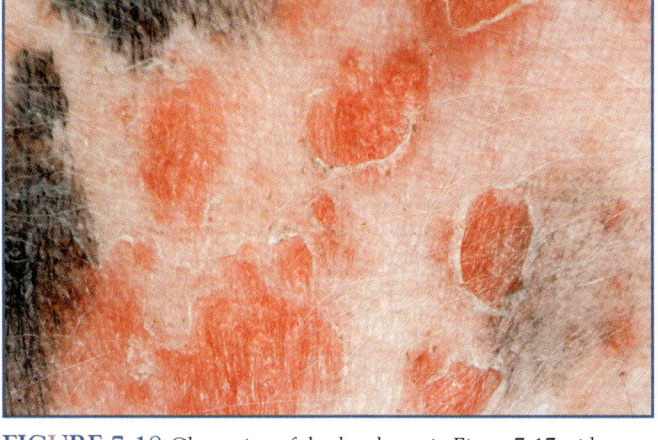

FIGURE 7-18 *Closer view of the dog shown in Figure 7-17 with superficial spreading pyoderma. Coalescing collarettes have formed large, irregular erythematous rings. Older lesions leave residual hyperpigmentation as a sequela.*

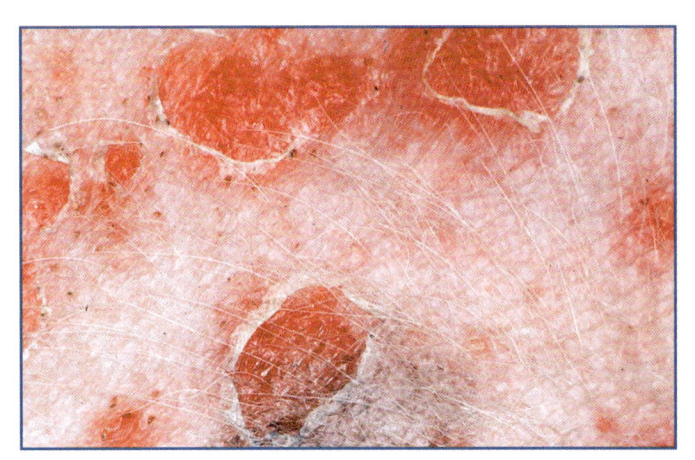

FIGURE 7-19 *An additional closer view of the dog seen in Figure 7-17 with superficial spreading pyoderma. Minimal folliculitis is present.*

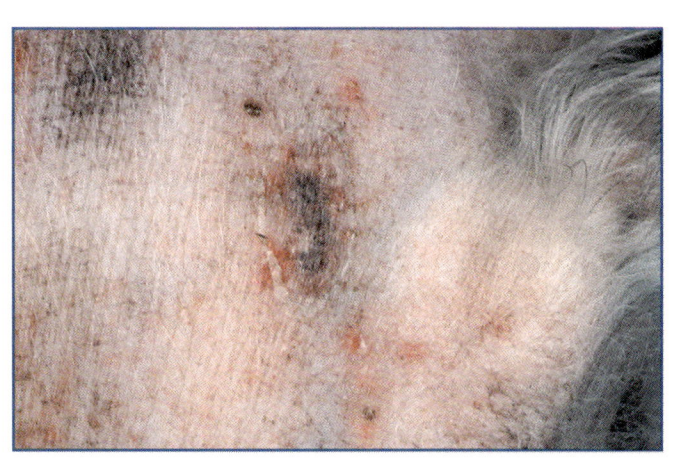

FIGURE 7-20 *Superficial spreading pyoderma in an adult cocker spaniel–poodle crossbreed. Postinflammatory hyperpigmentation is present centrally. (Courtesy of Dr. Carlo Vitale, case material, University of California.)*

at the margins of the expanding macules as the superficial keratin layer lifts and peels peripherally. Central crusting may be present. As expanding macules impinge on each other, irregular arciform patterns develop, resembling the interconnecting ripples seen when multiple stones are dropped into still water.

After inflammation subsides, postinflammatory hyperpigmentation marks the site of previously active lesions (Figure 7-20). If inflammation is substantial, alopecia may occur in ringlike patterns within the confines of the macules. Pruritus is quite variable but usually is present. Surprisingly, pruritus may not correlate with the magnitude of erythema. The glabrous skin of the ventrum is most commonly affected, but lesions may generalize on the trunk (Figure 7-21).

Signalment Predilections

Breed, age, or sex predilections have not been reported. Superficial spreading pyoderma is seen in many breeds of dogs. Border collies, Australian shepherds, and Shetland sheepdogs may be predisposed to exceptionally florid lesions. A particularly striking subgroup of combined superficial spreading pyoderma and superficial folliculitis is seen in Shetland sheepdogs, whereby infection leads to large coalescing areas of lateral truncal alopecia with scaling and

FIGURE 7-16 *Superficial spreading pyoderma. (1) Expanding coalescing erythematous rings with well-demarcated peripheral scaling collarette. (2) Peripheral collarette. (3) Bacteria dissect the layers of the stratum corneum, creating the collarette.*

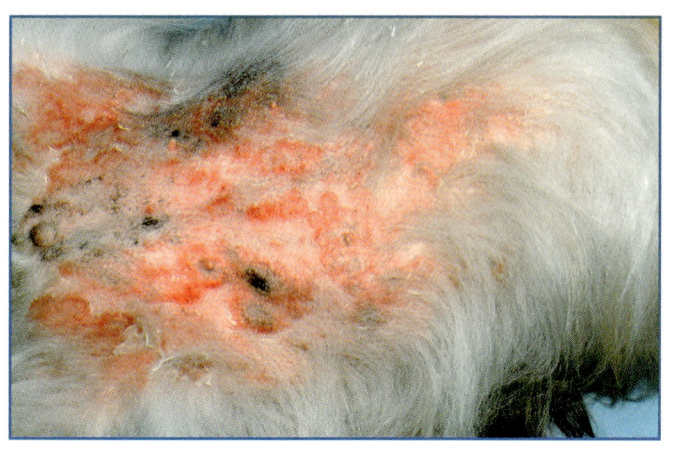

FIGURE 7-21 *Superficial spreading pyoderma on the ventral abdomen of a Shetland sheepdog. Inflammation and pruritus were exceptionally severe. (Courtesy of Dr. Alexander Werner, case material, University of California.)*

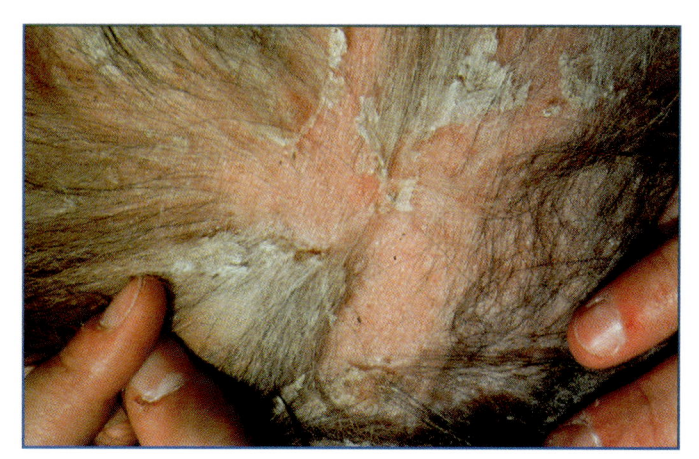

FIGURE 7-22 *Combined superficial folliculitis and superficial spreading pyoderma in a Shetland sheepdog. Large coalescing rings of alopecia have formed on the lateral thorax.*

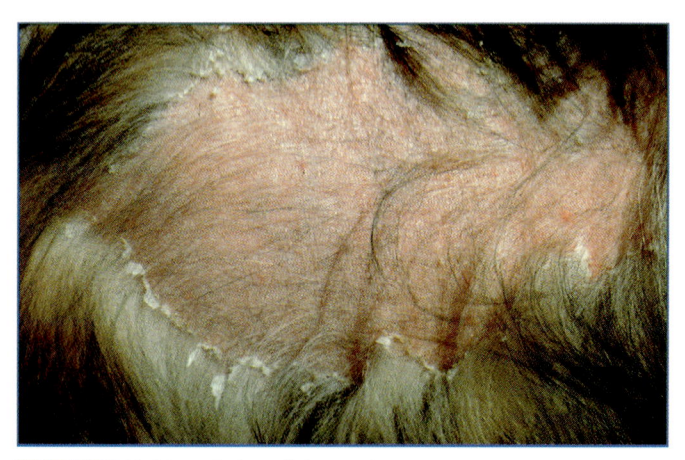

FIGURE 7-23 *Right lateral thorax of the Shetland sheepdog in Figure 7-22 with combined superficial folliculitis and superficial spreading pyoderma. Coalescing rings of alopecia have led to the formation of an alopecic patch involving most of the lateral thorax.*

hyperpigmentation (Figures 7-22 and 7-23). Individual alopecic patches may exceed 15 cm in diameter.

Differential Diagnosis and Diagnosis

Clinical diagnostic differentials for lesions with obvious peripheral epidermal collarettes include superficial bacterial folliculitis, pemphigus foliaceus, erythema multiforme, and sterile eosinophilic pustulosis. Superficial bacterial folliculitis is unlikely as a principal diagnosis if either pustules or focal, crusted papules are sparse. Although early erythema multiforme may resemble superficial spreading pyoderma, erythema usually extends well beyond the confines of the epidermal collarette, and erosions or ulceration usually occur within several days after lesions form. Localization of lesions to the ventrum would be exceedingly unusual for canine pemphigus foliaceus. Sterile eosinophilic pustulosis is a very rare disease characterized by marked pruritus and pustules. If pruritus and attendant self-trauma are marked, lesions may be considerably less diagnostic and may resemble flea allergy dermatitis or dermatophytosis.

Diagnosis is accomplished by history, clinical signs, distribution of lesions, and, commonly, response to appropriate therapy. Skin biopsy of the advancing edge of the epidermal collarette is confirmatory. Biopsy of the central region of the erythematous macules is less likely to yield diagnostic results. When performing the skin biopsy, care should be taken not to dislodge the scale present at the margin of the epidermal collarette because this material is most likely to yield a definitive diagnosis. If pustules are present, they also should be sampled.

Skin biopsy reveals small, loosely organized, spongiotic, superficial epidermal pustules as the most characteristic lesions. Gram-positive cocci accompanied by granular basophilic debris may be seen within the superficial layers of the stratum corneum. This mixture of bacteria and basophilic debris has been referred to as "Dunstan's blue line."[7] The lifting of keratin that is sometimes evident above or adjacent to the blue line probably corresponds to the epidermal collarette seen clinically. Superficial, predominantly neutrophilic dermal inflammation is present.[7]

Therapeutic Overview and Prognosis

Superficial spreading pyoderma is a common canine bacterial skin disease that may either be seen alone or coexist with canine superficial bacterial folliculitis. Response to appropriate therapy is rapid, but recrudescence is common if therapy is discontinued before complete clinical cure is achieved. Recurrent superficial spreading pyoderma may be frustrating to treat, similar to recurrent superficial bacterial folliculitis. Recurrence indicates the need to pursue the possibility of underlying predisposing factors such as allergic diseases.

Systemic antibiotic therapy is necessary to achieve clinical remission in dogs with superficial spreading pyoderma. A minimum of 3 to 4 weeks of appropriate systemic antibiotic therapy is recommended (see Chapter 10). Systemic antibiotics should be continued for an additional 2 weeks beyond clinical cure.

Adjunctive topical therapy is strongly recommended. Antibacterial shampoos may be particularly useful because infection occurs between the layers of the stratum corneum; therefore, shampooing may remove the nidus of possible future infection. As in superficial bacterial folliculitis, benefits may include enhanced speed of recovery and diminished likelihood of recurrence as well as improvement in patient attitude.[18,19] Clinical impression suggests that antibacterial shampoos may have long-term benefits in diminishing the likelihood of recurrence.[20]

Potentially beneficial antibacterial shampoos include those containing benzoyl peroxide and sulfur,[d] benzoyl peroxide,[e–g] ethyl lactate,[c] and chlorhexidine.[b] Initially, the entire dog should be bathed. Weekly bathing of the entire dog can be supplemented with cleansing of the affected area between the weekly shampoos. If recurrence without identifiable underlying causes manifests, weekly antibacterial shampoos can be used in an attempt to diminish the frequency of recrudescence.

> Systemic antibiotic therapy is necessary to achieve clinical remission in dogs with superficial spreading pyoderma.

[a]Bactoderm®, Pfizer Animal Health.
[b]ChlorhexiDerm, DVM Pharmaceuticals.
[c]Etiderm™, Allerderm/Virbac.
[d]Sulf/OxyDex, DVM Pharmaceuticals.
[e]Pyoben®, Allerderm/Virbac.
[f]OxyDex, DVM Pharmaceuticals.
[g]Micro Pearls™ Benzoyl Peroxide Shampoo, Evsco Pharmaceuticals.

REFERENCES

1. Ihrke PJ, Halliwell REW, Deubler MJ: Canine pyoderma, in Kirk RW (ed): *Current Veterinary Therapy VI*. Philadelphia, WB Saunders, 1976, pp 513–519.
2. Ihrke PJ: The management of canine pyodermas, in Kirk RW (ed): *Current Veterinary Therapy VIII*. Philadelphia, WB Saunders, 1983, pp 505–517.
3. Ihrke PJ: An overview of bacterial skin disease in the dog. *Br Vet J* 433:112–118, 1987.
4. White SD, Ihrke PJ: Pyoderma, in Nesbitt GH (ed): *Dermatology—Contemporary Issues in Small Animal Practice*. New York, Churchill Livingstone, 1987, pp 95–121.
5. Fourrier P, Carlotti D, Magnol J-P: Les pyodermites superficielles. *Prat Med Chirurg Anim Compag* 23:473–484, 1988.
6. Ihrke PJ: Bacterial infections of the skin, in Greene CE (ed): *Infectious Diseases of the Dog and Cat*. Philadelphia, WB Saunders, 1990, pp 72–79.
7. Gross TL, Ihrke PJ, Walder EJ: *Veterinary Dermatopathology: A Macroscopic and Microscopic Evaluation of Canine and Feline Skin Disease*. St. Louis, Mosby–Year Book, 1992, pp 10–14, 238–240, 252–255.
8. Mason I: Pustules and crusted papules, in Locke PH, Harvey RG, Mason IS (eds): *Manual of Small Animal Dermatology*. Gloucestershire, BSAVA, 1993, pp 60–64.
9. Scott DW, Miller WH, Griffin CE: *Muller & Kirk's Small Animal Dermatology*, ed 5. Philadelphia, WB Saunders, 1995, pp 279–328.
10. Sisco WM, Ihrke PJ, Franti CE: Regional distribution of the common skin diseases in dogs. *JAVMA* 195:752–756, 1989.
11. Ihrke PJ: Global veterinary dermatology, in Parish LC, Millikan LE, Amer M, et al (eds): *Global Dermatology: Diagnosis and Management According to Geography, Climate, and Culture*. New York, Springer-Verlag, 1995, pp 103–110.
12. Ihrke PJ, Schwartzman RM, McGinley K, et al: Microbiology of normal and seborrheic canine skin. *Am J Vet Res* 39:1487–1489, 1978.
13. Mason IS, Lloyd DH: The role of allergy in the development of canine pyoderma. *J Small Anim Pract* 30:216–218, 1989.
14. Mason IS: Hypersensitivity and the multiplication of staphylococci on canine skin (PhD thesis). London, University of London, 1990, pp 1–172.
15. Horwitz LN, Ihrke PJ: Canine seborrhea, in Kirk RW (ed): *Current Veterinary Therapy VI*. Philadelphia, WB Saunders, 1976, pp 519–524.
16. Kristensen S, Krogh HV: A study of skin diseases in dogs and cats—III. Microflora of the skin of dogs with chronic eczema. *Nord Vet Med* 30:223–230, 1978.
17. McEwan NA: Bacterial adherence to canine corneocytes, in Von Tscharner C, Halliwell REW (eds): *Advances in Veterinary Dermatology*, vol 1. London, Baillière Tindall, 1990, p 454.
18. Lloyd DH, Reyss-Brion DA: Le peroxyde de benzoyle: Efficacite clinique et bacteriologique dans le traitement des pyodermites chroniques. *Prat Med Chirurg Anim Compag* 19(6):445–449, 1984.
19. Ihrke PJ: Antibacterial therapy in dermatology, in Kirk RW (ed): *Current Veterinary Therapy IX*. Philadelphia, WB Saunders, 1986, pp 566–571.
20. Ihrke PJ, Gross TL: Clinico-pathologic conferences in dermatology—#1: Superficial spreading pyoderma. *Vet Dermatol* 4(1):33–36, 1994.

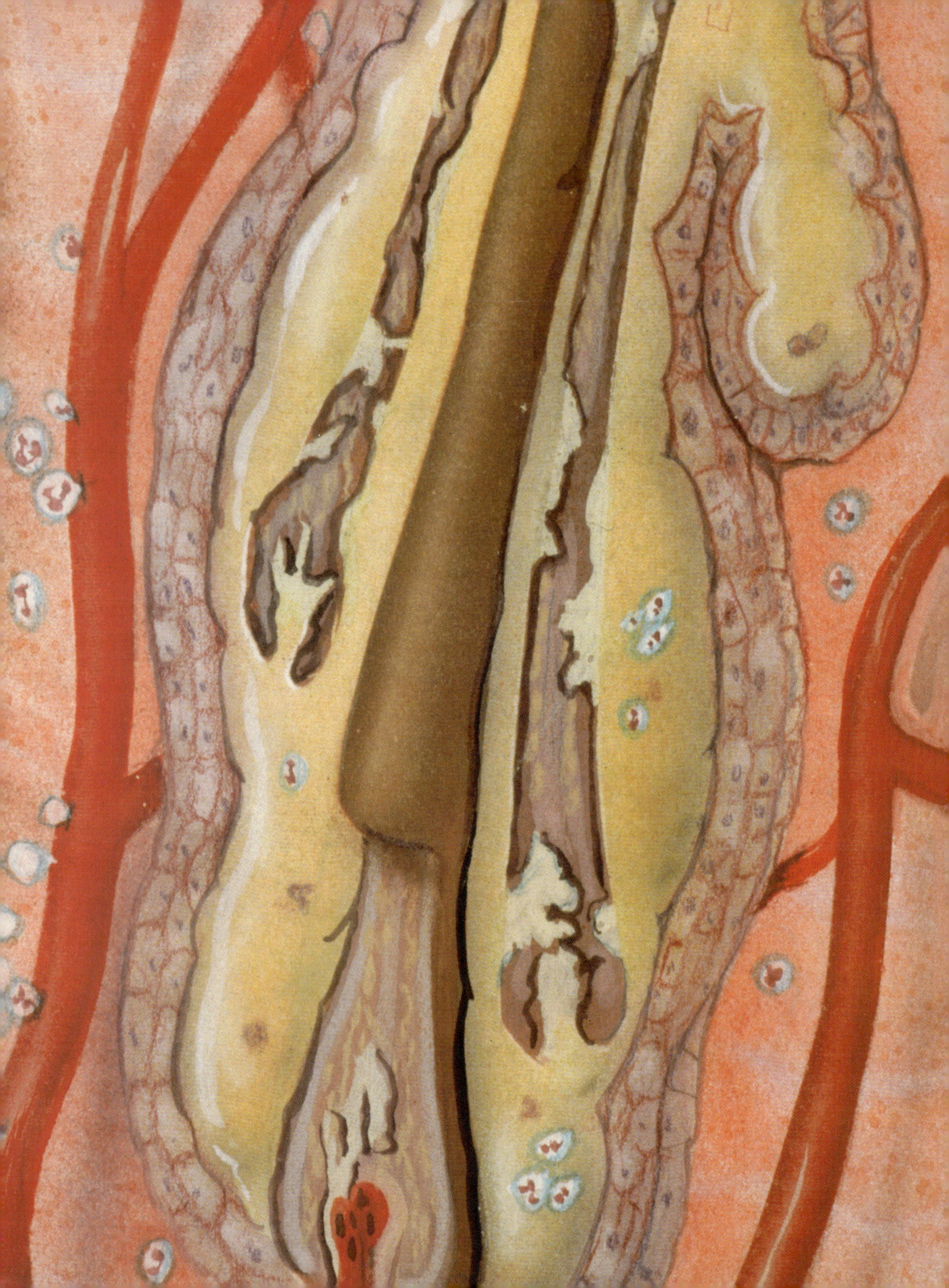

Chapter 8

Deep Pyoderma

DEEP BACTERIAL FOLLICULITIS AND FURUNCULOSIS

General Considerations

Deep bacterial folliculitis and furunculosis is seen less commonly than superficial bacterial folliculitis but is still a relatively common canine bacterial skin disease[1-5] (Figure 8-1). The pathogenesis of deep bacterial folliculitis and furunculosis is controversial. It may develop de novo without evidence of prior superficial folliculitis or occur as a progression from superficial folliculitis. The mechanisms by which some follicular infections remain in the ostial portion of the hair follicle, some proceed downward, and others immediately affect the entire follicular canal are unknown.[5] Deep follicular inflammation commonly leads to follicular rupture and, hence, furunculosis. A granulomatous foreign body response directed against free keratin from the root sheath and hair shaft fragments fosters the formation of scar tissue with sequestered pyogranulomas. Consequentially, the dual problems of infection and foreign body granulomas coexist.[5,6]

Staphylococcus intermedius is the primary pathogen, as is the case in all other canine pyodermas. However, in deep pyoderma, secondary invaders such as *Proteus*, *Pseudomonas*, and *Escherichia coli* are seen more frequently than in other canine pyodermas.

Most cases of deep pyoderma have an underlying cause. As discussed in Chapter 3, any inflammatory, obstructive, atrophic, dysplastic, or degenerative disease of the hair follicle can predispose dogs to secondary bacterial infection. Diminished or altered immune surveillance may predispose them to deeper infection. Deep pyoderma is common secondary to demodicosis. Naturally occurring hyperadrenocorticism or the injudicious use of glucocorticoids (iatrogenic hyperglucocorticoidism) also predisposes dogs to deeper infection. In addition, follicular obstructive diseases such as calluses, actinic comedones, and schnauzer comedo syndrome also predispose dogs to deep pyoderma.[5,6]

Occasionally, direct follicular trauma can be the inciting cause of furunculosis by causing traumatic implantation of hair shafts beyond the confines of the hair follicle and into the surrounding dermis. Owners or groomers may induce traumatic furunculosis by close clipping "against the grain" (against the direction of hair coat growth) or even by aggressive "back combing."[5] Traumatic furunculosis can also be self-induced by the dog. Persistent licking in cases of acral lick dermatitis can induce traumatic follicular rupture, and pressure applied to bony prominences by reclining on hard surfaces can initiate follicular rupture and cause callus pyoderma.

Clinical Findings

As in superficial bacterial folliculitis, inflammatory pustules center around hair follicles. The pustules of deep bacterial folliculitis and furunculosis tend to be larger. If multiple hair follicles are involved, but the infection does not involve all neighboring follicles, the erythematous bases of the pustules are visible as discrete, firm nodules (Figure 8-2). If infection becomes confluent, involving large groups of hair follicles in a region, poorly defined edematous plaques form and individual pustules and nodules are less obvious (Figures 8-3 and 8-4).

Pus from intact pustules or draining from fistulas varies in color from white to yellow-grey. A change in the hue of pus to pink or red signifies the presence

> In deep pyoderma, secondary invaders such as *Proteus*, *Pseudomonas*, and *Escherichia coli* are seen more frequently than in other canine pyodermas.

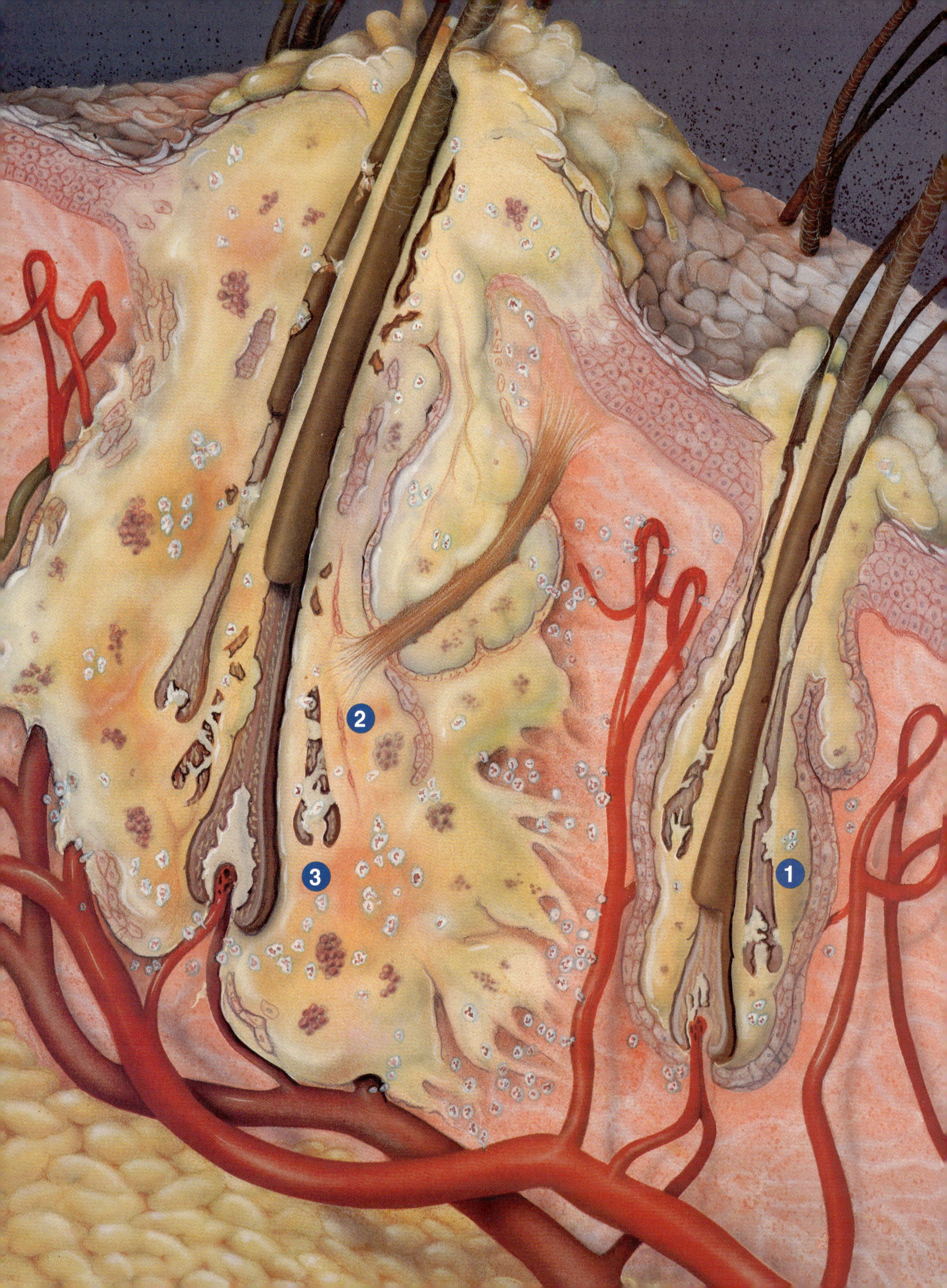

1
2
3

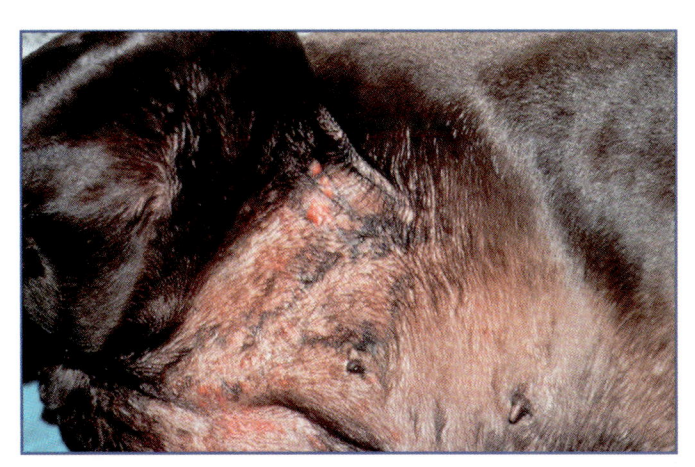

FIGURE 8-2 *Deep bacterial folliculitis and furunculosis on the ventral abdomen of a dog. Note the pustules and erythematous raised nodules.*

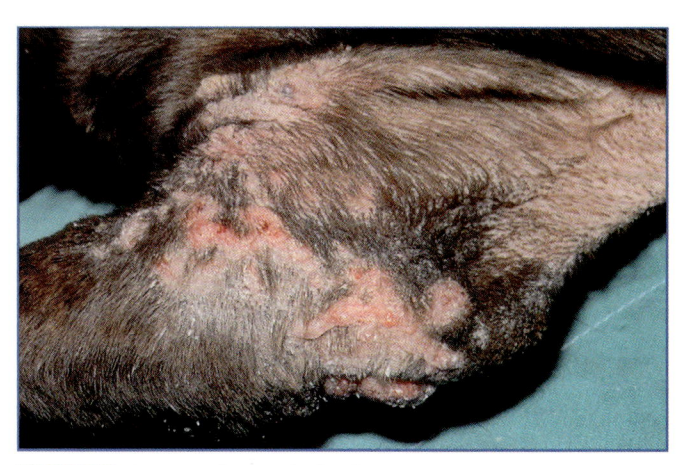

FIGURE 8-3 *Deep bacterial folliculitis and furunculosis in the axillary region of a beagle crossbreed. Note that infection is becoming confluent as nodules coalesce.*

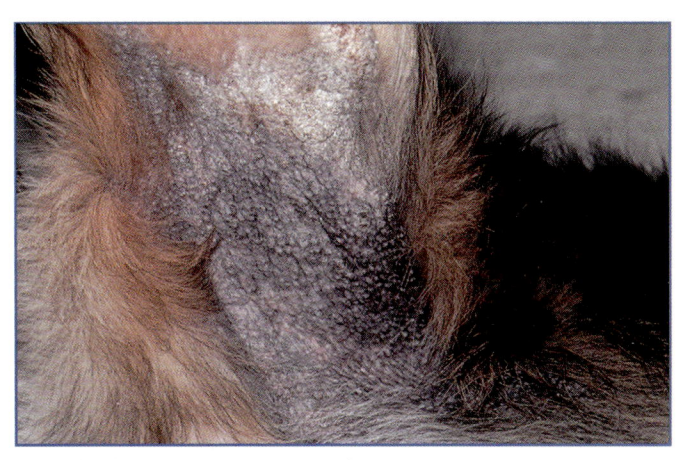

FIGURE 8-4 *Deep bacterial folliculitis and furunculosis in the axillary region of a German shepherd. The infection has become confluent as individual lesions are less obvious.*

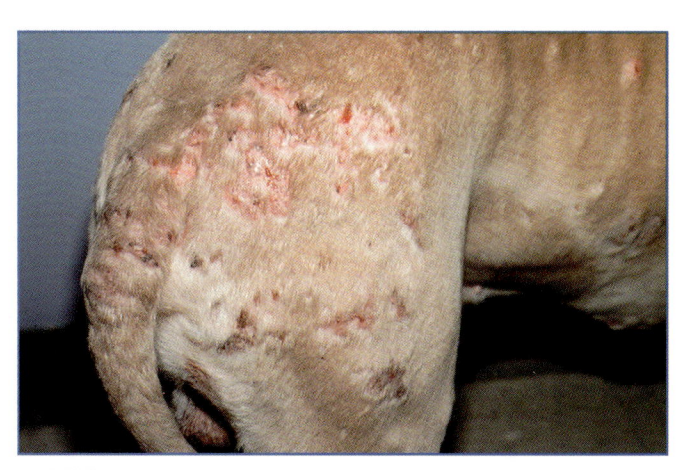

FIGURE 8-5 *Generalized deep bacterial folliculitis and furunculosis in a bullterrier. Multiple areas of infection are obvious in this short-coated dog.*

of hemorrhage, indicating more severe dermal damage. Pustules, discrete nodules, and edematous plaques ulcerate, which leads to draining fistulas or less diagnostic hemorrhagic crusts. Frank surface necrosis may be seen in areas of more confluent infection. Hyperpigmentation and lichenification occur with chronicity. As in superficial infection, follicular inflammation and destruction lead to varying degrees of alopecia. Lesions are more visually obvious in short-coated dogs (Figure 8-5). In long-coated dogs, debris matted in the hair coat may shield severe lesions from view until the affected area is clipped.

Pain or pruritus commonly is present. Lymphadenopathy usually is present and may be regional or generalized. Additional constitutional signs may be seen and are contingent on the severity and extent of deep pyoderma and any underlying disease.

Hemorrhagic bullae are an additional distinctive clinical feature of deep pyoderma in some dogs.[5,6] Slightly raised, firm nodules or plaques vary in color from red to dark blue or violet (Figures 8-6 to 8-8). Diascopy (i.e., placing a glass slide firmly against the skin to ascertain whether erythema can be blanched) reveals that the red blood cells are extravascular, which indicates hemorrhage. Hemorrhagic lesions that are more recent and fresh tend to be brighter red. Occasionally, erythematous, hemorrhagic rings may surround older lesions. These lesions have been seen in a variety of breeds but may be evident more frequently in the German shepherd, bullterrier, and

FIGURE 8-1 *Deep folliculitis and furunculosis. (1) Deep folliculitis (note the infection is within the confines of an intact hair follicle). (2) Furunculosis. The hair follicle has ruptured, spreading infection into the dermis. (3) Remnant of a hair shaft within the furuncle.*

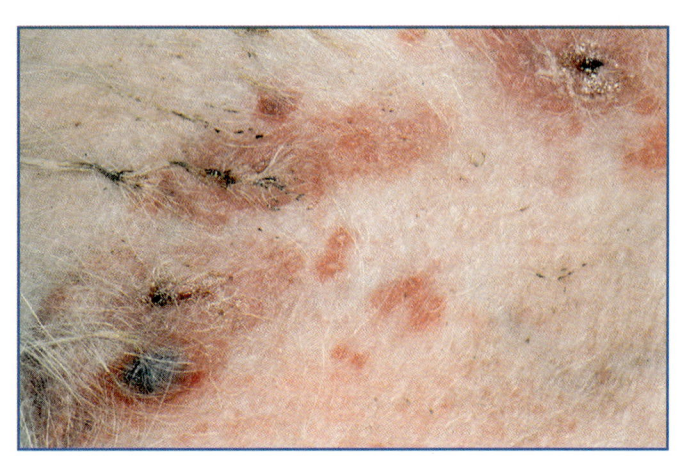

FIGURE 8-6 *Multiple pustules, nodules, and hemorrhagic bullae on the ventral abdomen of a dog with deep pyoderma.*

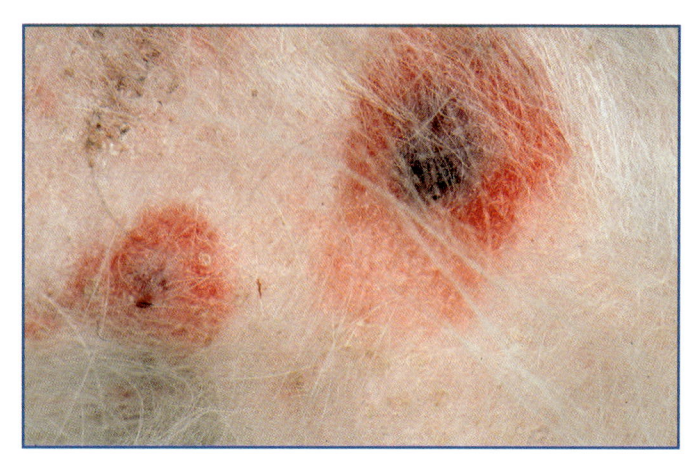

FIGURE 8-7 *Hemorrhagic bullae associated with deep pyoderma in the same dog seen in Figure 8-6.*

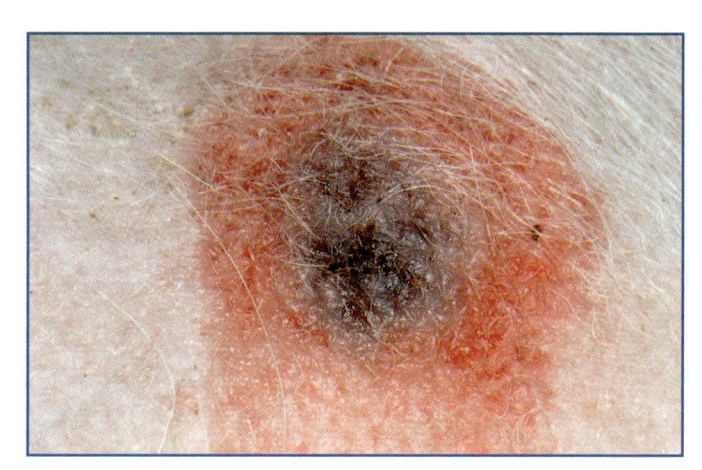

FIGURE 8-8 *Closer view of the lesion shown in Figure 8-7. Hemorrhage surrounds an indurated plaque of deep pyoderma.*

dalmatian.[5] Dogs with demodicosis and actinic comedones seem to be predisposed to the formation of hemorrhagic bullae.

Initial sites of involvement mirror those of superficial folliculitis. The intertriginous zones of the groin, axillae, and interdigital webs are commonly affected. As indicated above, deep pyoderma secondary to ruptured hair follicles occurs in canine callosities located over pressure points. Lesions may generalize, especially if the underlying predisposing cause is immunosuppression or demodicosis.

Certain types of deep bacterial folliculitis and furunculosis are clinically distinctive enough to warrant subdivision and individual discussion. However, the basic material discussed under the larger heading of deep bacterial folliculitis and furunculosis is still applicable. These syndromes include muzzle folliculitis and furunculosis (canine acne), pyotraumatic folliculitis, pedal folliculitis and furunculosis, callus pyoderma (pressure-point pyoderma), and German shepherd dog pyoderma. A syndrome termed *nasal folliculitis and furunculosis* (nasal pyoderma) is controversial.[6] The author believes that most of the dogs previously classified as having nasal pyoderma probably had eosinophilic folliculitis and furunculosis of the face due to arthropod hypersensitivity.[5,7]

Signalment Predilections

Breed, age, and sex predilections vary with specific subgroups of deep bacterial folliculitis and furunculosis. Among long-coated dogs, the German shepherd, golden retriever, and Irish setter may be predisposed to various deep pyodermas. According to Kwochka, chronic relapsing deep pyoderma is more common in short-coated breeds, possibly due to a more intense foreign body reaction to keratin.[8] Short-coated dogs at apparent increased risk include the bullterrier breeds, dalmatian, Doberman pinscher, and Great Dane.[5] Deep pyoderma secondary to demodicosis obviously follows the predilections of the underlying demodicosis. In general, sex predilections are not seen. Other generalizations applying to all subgroups cannot be made.

Differential Diagnosis and Diagnosis

General clinical diagnostic differentials for deep bacterial folliculitis and furunculosis include demodicosis with or without a secondary bacterial component, subcutaneous and deep mycoses, opportunistic fungal infections, severe maladapted dermatophytosis, sterile granuloma/pyogranuloma, histiocytosis, idiopathic nodular panniculitis, juvenile sterile granulomatous dermatitis and lymphadenitis (juvenile cellulitis), vasculitis, and pythiosis (Table 8-1).

TABLE 8-1
GENERAL CLINICAL DIAGNOSTIC DIFFERENTIALS FOR DEEP BACTERIAL FOLLICULITIS AND FURUNCULOSIS

- Demodicosis with or without a secondary bacterial component
- Subcutaneous and deep mycoses
- Opportunistic fungal infections
- Severe maladapted dermatophytosis
- Sterile granuloma/pyogranuloma
- Histiocytosis
- Idiopathic nodular panniculitis
- Juvenile sterile granulomatous dermatitis and lymphadenitis (juvenile cellulitis)
- Vasculitis
- Pythiosis

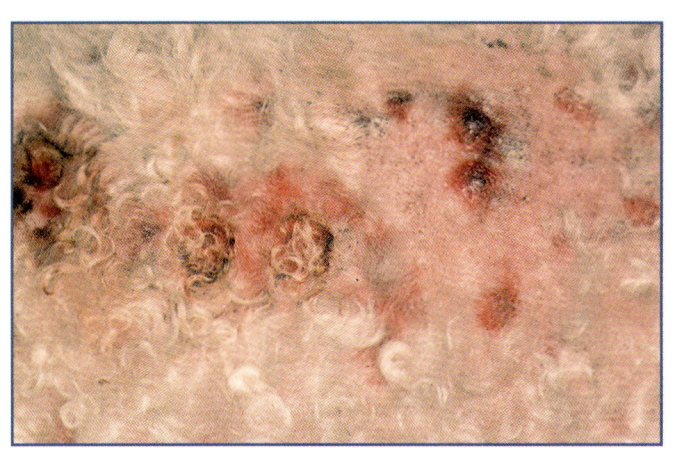

FIGURE 8-9 *Deep pyoderma with prominent hemorrhagic bullae secondary to sebaceous adenitis in a white standard poodle.*

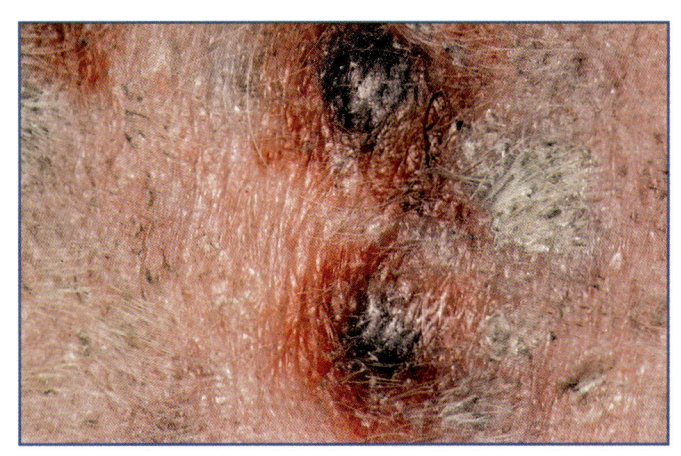

FIGURE 8-10 *Closer view of hemorrhagic bullae with sebaceous adenitis in the standard poodle seen in Figure 8-9.*

Differentiation is accomplished by skin scrapings (to rule out underlying demodicosis), microscopic examination of stained smears of exudates (to evaluate for the presence of and identify pathogenic organisms), histopathology, and, possibly, bacterial and fungal cultures. Skin biopsy recommendations and histopathologic findings are similar for most deep pyodermas and are reviewed here. Greater detail with respect to other diagnostic findings are provided below as each subgroup is discussed.

Whenever possible, early lesions should be sampled for skin biopsy. Contingent on the lesions present, intact pustules, nodules, hemorrhagic bullae, or erythematous, edematous plaques may be sampled. Older, scarred lesions are less likely to yield diagnostic follicular lesions but may be useful as prognosticators.

The principal histopathologic features of deep bacterial folliculitis and furunculosis are neutrophilic inflammation within the follicular wall and canal, follicular rupture, and furuncle formation. Follicles may be completely effaced and replaced by nodular mixed inflammation (neutrophils and macrophages located centrally and plasma cells located peripherally) and scar tissue. Free hair shafts and other fragments of follicular debris may be present at the center of pyogranulomas. Lesions may extend into the panniculus. Hemorrhagic bullae consist of large hemorrhagic pustules. It is not understood why these lesions may spare hair follicles and localize in an interfollicular location. Scarring may be severe.[5]

Therapeutic Overview and Prognosis

Deep bacterial folliculitis and furunculosis frequently eventuates from superficial bacterial folliculitis; therefore, much of the information discussed for the therapeutic management of superficial folliculitis is also applicable to the management of deep pyoderma. The identification and management of underlying causes are crucial to the successful treatment of deep bacterial folliculitis and furunculosis (Figures 8-9 and 8-10). Requisite therapy and prognosis vary widely; however, certain generalizations can be made. Systemic antibiotic therapy always is required for the successful management of deep pyoderma, with the exception of very mild cases of muzzle folliculitis and furunculosis (canine acne). A minimum of 4 to 6 weeks of systemic antibiotic therapy is required for successful management. In general, systemic antibiotics should be continued for a minimum of at least 2 weeks beyond apparent clinical cure in all cases of deep pyoderma because sequestered foci of infection often remain after most lesions have cleared.

Adjunctive topical therapy (as well as antibacterial soaks and whirlpools) is always beneficial, including antibacterial shampoos such as those discussed in Chapters 7 and 10. Clipping may be necessary in long-coated dogs if proper cleansing and drainage is impeded by the hair coat. The entire dog should be bathed, although efforts may be concentrated on severely affected areas. Dogs with deep pyoderma should be bathed at least weekly and preferably twice weekly.

Antibacterial soaks and whirlpools are used too infrequently in veterinary medicine and are extremely beneficial in the management of deep pyoderma. Chlorhexidine or povidone-iodine solution is added to warm water (see Chapter 10). Hospitalization and antibacterial whirlpools or soaks once or twice daily are strongly recommended. Profound improvement in patient attitude and owner encouragement are additional benefits.

MUZZLE FOLLICULITIS AND FURUNCULOSIS (CANINE ACNE)

General Considerations

Muzzle folliculitis and furunculosis, commonly known as canine acne, is a common, chronic, inflammatory skin disease seen predominantly in prepubescent and pubescent dogs. The condition is characterized clinically by the formation of comedones (blackheads) on the chin and lips. Characteristic bacterial furuncles are seen secondary to an initial apparently sterile follicular inflammatory process. Previously, it has been hypothesized that, similar to human acne, increased production of androgens may induce increased production of sebum leading to inflammation and comedo formation.[9] Recently, Scott, Miller, and Griffin have speculated that "local trauma and possibly some undetermined genetic predisposition" are central to the pathogenesis of this syndrome and that rough play in short-coated puppies causes short hairs to break off below the skin surface, which subsequently initiates a sterile inflammatory process that leads to secondary bacterial invasion.[6] The observations that muzzle folliculitis and furunculosis is seen in intact or neutered males and female dogs with apparently equal frequency, and almost exclusively in short-coated dogs, do not support the older theory that excess androgen production leads to this syndrome.[6]

Clinical Findings

Erythematous follicular papules give rise to pustules, crusted papules, and comedones (Figure 8-11). Comedones on raised erythematous bases contain dark, inspissated follicular debris. Loss of hair from affected follicles can lead to extensive localized alopecia. Follicular perforation results in the formation of firm nodules, furuncles, fistulous tracts, and alopecia. Extensive scarring develops with chronicity.

The most common sites for canine muzzle folliculitis and furunculosis include the rostral portion of the chin and the skin surrounding the lower lips. The region above the upper lips and the lateral muzzle are also affected in more severe cases. Partial bilateral symmetry is noted. Pruritus is variable and, when present, usually is mild. Pain occurs in more severe cases.

Signalment Predilections

Muzzle folliculitis and furunculosis is seen almost exclusively in short-coated breeds. The Doberman pinscher, Great Dane, English bulldog, German shorthaired pointer, boxer, mastiff, rottweiler, and weimaraner appear to be overrepresented.[5,6] Disease onset usually coincides with puberty, and dogs between 5 and 12 months of age are affected most frequently. The syndrome usually resolves spontaneously during young adulthood, but some cases persist. Sex predilections have not been noted.[5]

Differential Diagnosis and Diagnosis

Canine muzzle folliculitis and furun-

> In general, systemic antibiotics should be continued for a minimum of at least 2 weeks beyond apparent clinical cure in all cases of deep pyoderma because sequestered foci of infection often remain after most lesions have cleared.

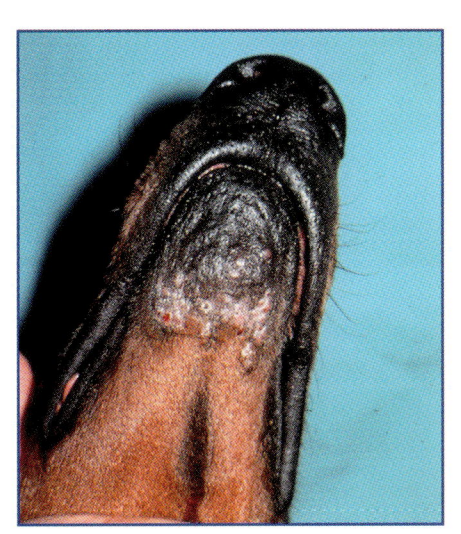

FIGURE 8-11
Canine muzzle folliculitis and furunculosis on the chin of a 7-month-old male Doberman pinscher. This deep pyoderma is seen commonly in young short-coated breeds.

culosis is visually distinctive. Most likely diagnostic differentials include localized demodicosis as well as early juvenile sterile granulomatous dermatitis and lymphadenitis (juvenile cellulitis). On occasion, dermatophytosis may be an additional differential diagnosis.

Tentative diagnosis is accomplished by deep skin scrapings (to rule out demodicosis) and, if deemed necessary, fungal culture. Lack of systemic signs aids in differentiating this syndrome from juvenile sterile granulomatous dermatitis and lymphadenitis (juvenile cellulitis). Response to therapy substantiates the diagnosis.

Skin biopsy is not performed routinely in the diagnosis of canine muzzle folliculitis and furunculosis because the lesions are highly characteristic visually. If substantiation of the diagnosis by skin biopsy is desired, the ventral chin is recommended as a cosmetically advantageous site. Punch biopsy sampling of larger comedones also may facilitate healing by removing severely affected hair follicles.

Diagnostic histopathologic findings include severe follicular keratosis and comedo formation. Intact comedones are surrounded by mixed inflammation. Ruptured comedones are characterized by severe inflammation and scarring.[5]

Therapeutic Overview and Prognosis

The aggressiveness of therapy is dictated by the severity and chronicity of the lesions. Topical antibacterial therapy is universally recommended. In early cases, topical corticosteroids may be beneficial. Severely affected dogs with extensive scarring will benefit from systemic antibiotics. Based on their hypothesis on the role of local trauma, Scott, Miller, and Griffin have recommended "modifications of behavior that traumatize the chin."[6]

Shampoos that contain benzoyl peroxide are recommended because of their combination of antibacterial and follicular flushing effect. Daily gentle cleansing of the affected area is recommended initially. As improvement is noted after 1 to 2 weeks, the frequency of cleansing can be reduced to every other day. Although gels containing benzoyl peroxide are available and frequently recommended in the management of this disease, the author usually does not recommend their use because the residue may bleach fabrics.

Systemic antibiotics are indicated in more severe cases of canine muzzle folliculitis and furunculosis that are characterized by fistulas and scarring. In milder cases, antibiotics can also be used to reduce the likelihood of scarring while topical therapy is diminishing inflammation. Systemic antibiotics should be used for a minimum of 4 to 6 weeks in the management of severe cases.

Patients with very mild, early cases of canine muzzle folliculitis and furunculosis may respond to topical corticosteroids. In addition, topical corticosteroids have been used to diminish inflammation as an adjunct to systemic antibiotics in more severe cases with marked scar tissue formation.[6] A topical antibiotic preparation containing mupirocin[a] can be applied to affected areas after an antibacterial shampoo and has been beneficial in a limited number of cases.

PYOTRAUMATIC FOLLICULITIS
General Considerations

The term *pyotraumatic folliculitis*[6] has been coined recently to refer to the focal or multifocal deep pyoderma that clinically can closely mimic the surface pyoderma pyotraumatic dermatitis. This syndrome was initially described as a

> The term *pyotraumatic folliculitis* has been coined recently to refer to the focal or multifocal deep pyoderma that clinically can closely mimic the surface pyoderma pyotraumatic dermatitis.

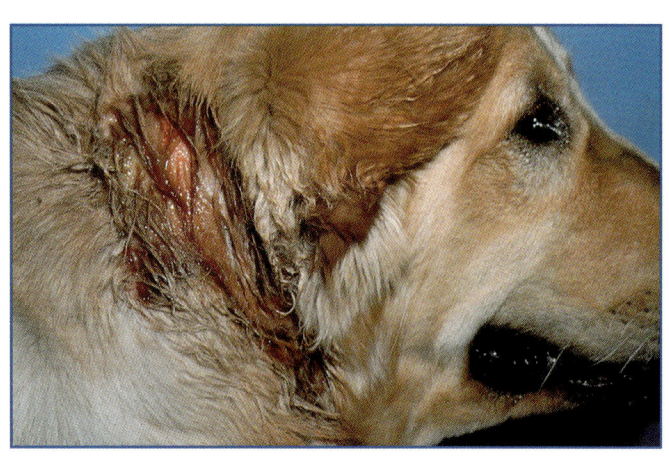

FIGURE 8-12 *Pyotraumatic folliculitis mimicking pyotraumatic dermatitis on the neck of a golden retriever. (Courtesy of Dr. Helen Power, case material, University of California.)*

clinically and histologically distinct subgroup of pyotraumatic dermatitis characterized by lesions typical of pyotraumatic dermatitis coupled with a subjacent deep folliculitis and furunculosis. Initially, it was hypothesized that deep pyoderma occurred secondary to the initial pyotraumatic dermatitis.[10] However, it is more likely that the syndrome begins with focal areas of painful or pruritic deep pyoderma that become secondarily severely self-traumatized, causing the creation of overlying surface lesions that clinically resemble pyotraumatic dermatitis.[3,5] It is not known why multifocal deep pyoderma, apparently without preexisting superficial pyoderma, occurs in this syndrome. Marked breed predilections, especially in the golden retriever, indicate a probable hereditary component. Underlying allergic disease is believed to be an additional risk factor. Recurrences are the rule rather than the exception with this disease.

Clinical Findings

The lesions of pyotraumatic folliculitis closely mimic those of pyotraumatic dermatitis. Sharply demarcated erythematous, slightly elevated plaques form in response to severe self-trauma (Figure 8-12). Self-trauma removes hair from the affected area, and exudative viscid debris mats the traumatically eroded or ulcerated lesion. Unlike pyotraumatic dermatitis, satellite lesions are common and may begin simply as moderately well-demarcated erythematous macules or plaques beyond the traumatized margin of the central lesion before self-trauma is initiated. Erythematous collarettes may sometimes be seen with early satellite lesions before obliterative self-trauma occurs. Pain or pruritus is similar to that in pyotraumatic folliculitis and pyotraumatic dermatitis. Perceptive owners may note focal discomfiture prior to the initiation of self-trauma and thus be able to predict the development of pyotraumatic folliculitis. The author knows of one owner who could reliably predict recurrent episodes when her dog shied away from the use of an obedience training collar.

Lesions are typically multifocal. The cheek and neck are common sites of involvement, but lesions may be seen elsewhere on the face and trunk. Lesions are *not* located on the dorsal lumbosacral region as is seen in pyotraumatic dermatitis secondary to flea allergy dermatitis.

Signalment Predilections

Pyotraumatic folliculitis occurs most frequently in the golden retriever and Saint Bernard but also is seen in other long-coated breeds such as the Newfoundland and Bernese mountain dog. The Labrador retriever may also be at increased risk.[5,10] Younger dogs seem preferentially affected.[10]

Differential Diagnosis and Diagnosis

Pyotraumatic dermatitis is the major differential diagnosis. Additionally, demodicosis, neoplasia (especially sweat gland adenocarcinoma), cutaneous metastasis, fixed drug eruptions, early necrotizing forms of idiopathic nodular panniculitis, early localized vasculitis, and focal *Malassezia* dermatitis or candidiasis are other substantially less likely diagnostic differentials.

Pyotraumatic folliculitis usually can be differentiated from pyotraumatic dermatitis based on history, number of lesions, satellite lesions, and site predilections. Consideration of pyotraumatic folliculitis or any of the other diagnostic differential mentioned above is warranted in a dog with pyotraumatic dermatitis that does not respond to appropriate empiric therapy. Diagnosis is confirmed by skin biopsy. Histopathologic lesions include features of pyotraumatic dermatitis overlying those of deep bacterial folliculitis and furunculosis.

Therapeutic Overview and Prognosis

Pyotraumatic folliculitis, especially in

> Recurrence after apparently successful therapy is common in cases of pyotraumatic folliculitis.

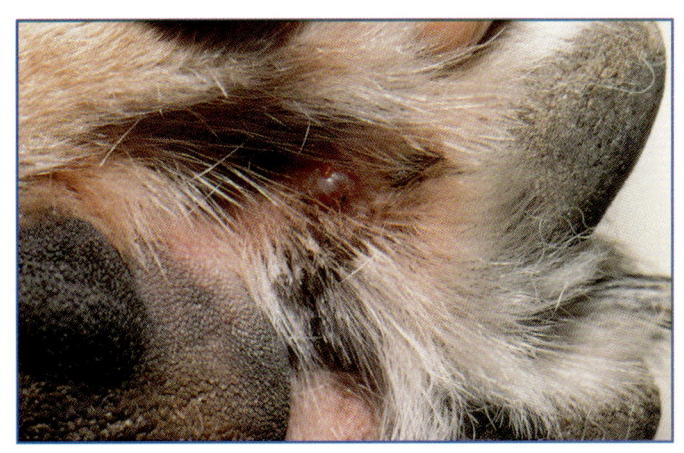

FIGURE 8-13 *Early pedal folliculitis and furunculosis in a mixed-breed dog. Note the discrete draining nodule. (Courtesy of Dr. Ralf Mueller, case material, University of California.)*

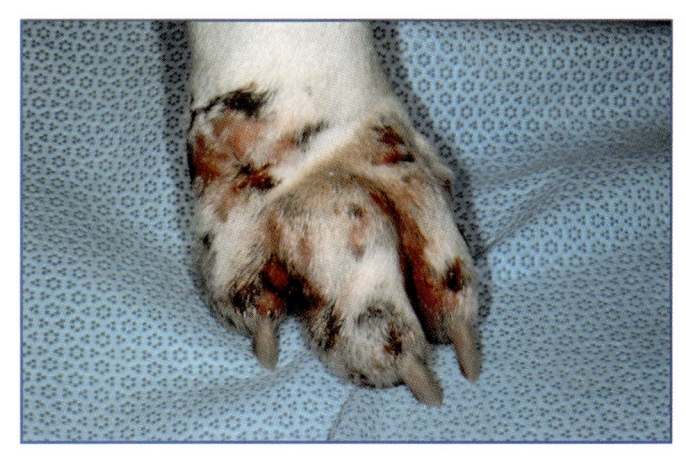

FIGURE 8-14 *Chronic pedal folliculitis and furunculosis in a boxer. Note that lesions are both interdigital and digital. (Courtesy of Dr. Ann Hargis, case material, University of California.)*

the golden retriever, is rarely a solitary event. Recurrence after apparently successful therapy is common. The duration of weeks to months between each episode indicates the likelihood that these are true recurrences rather than simply exacerbations following incomplete therapeutic success. Consequently, the identification and management of predisposing causes is crucial to the successful management of pyotraumatic folliculitis.

Underlying allergic diseases appear to be the primary trigger for pyotraumatic folliculitis. Both atopic dermatitis and food allergy probably predispose dogs to the development of this syndrome. Combined atopic dermatitis, food allergy, and flea allergy dermatitis have been noted as coexisting underlying causes in several golden retrievers! Management of predisposing causes plus additional recommendations to prevent recurrence (see Chapter 13) often are necessary.

Pyotraumatic folliculitis is managed effectively with systemic antibiotics plus adjunctive therapy for the overlying pyotraumatic dermatitis (see Chapter 6). In general, systemic antibiotics should be given for 4 to 6 weeks. As with other types of deep pyoderma, systemic antibiotics should be continued for a minimum of at least 2 weeks beyond apparent clinical cure because sequestered foci of infection often remain after visible lesions have cleared.

> The term *pedal folliculitis and furunculosis* has recently been suggested as a replacement for the categorization of interdigital or digital pyoderma.

PEDAL FOLLICULITIS AND FURUNCULOSIS

General Considerations

Digital and interdigital inflammatory diseases are grouped by convention under the category of pododermatitis—a condition that is very common in the dog.[11] Classification and diagnosis are difficult because, with chronicity, pododermatitis due to varied underlying causes can look very similar visually. Compounding diagnostic difficulties, pyoderma commonly complicates most other causes of digital and interdigital inflammatory disease in the dog.

Pyoderma is one of the most common causes of chronic pododermatitis.[6,11] The term *pedal folliculitis and furunculosis* has recently been suggested as a replacement for the categorization of interdigital or digital pyoderma.[6] This new terminology is beneficial because it takes into account that neither *digital* nor *interdigital* precisely delineates the location of all pedal bacterial infections. In addition, the new term specifies that this subgroup of pyoderma is always deep.

The reasons why distal extremities are such common sites for deep pyoderma are unclear. Certainly, the frequency of pedal self-trauma associated with allergic skin disease may be an initiating factor. In addition, the rather tight intertriginous spaces seen interdigitally in some dogs may encourage heat and moisture retention and foster bacterial overgrowth. In some breeds (notably short-coated dogs with stiff hair), follicular retention cysts that form interdigitally may rupture, initiating deep pyoderma.[12] Trauma is a likely contributory cause of interdigital lesions on the palmar surface of the feet. Hypothyroidism and Cushing's disease are other predisposing causes in addition to allergic diseases, trauma, and anatomic factors.[11]

Clinical Findings

Inflammatory pustules or firm nodules are likely to center around hair follicles. Initially, lesions tend to be discrete (Figure 8-13). Ulceration gives rise to draining fistulas (Figure 8-14). Scarring with ablation of the normal pedal architecture is noted with chronicity. Scar tissue formation may be dramatic. Early lesions tend to be haired, whereas alopecia is a feature of chronicity. Greater pain is associated with ventral interdigital involvement.

Lesions may be solitary but are usually multifocal. Poorly defined edematous plaques are more common when demodicosis is present as the underlying disease. Initial lesions develop interdigitally either on the plantar or palmar surface or on the digital skin on the plantar surface. Initially, interdigital lesions are more common than digital lesions.

Pedal folliculitis and furunculosis most commonly involves all four feet. The solitary involvement of just one foot enhances the likelihood of the presence of a foreign body or underlying neoplasia (especially squamous cell carcinoma or keratoacanthoma) as the initiating cause.

Signalment Predilections

Short-coated breeds such as the English bulldog, smooth-coated dachshund, boxer, Great Dane, mastiff, bullmastiff, bullterrier, basset hound, German shorthaired pointer, weimaraner, and dalmatian may be at greater risk. German shepherds, golden retrievers, Labrador retrievers, Pekingese, and Irish setters also are probably at increased risk. According to Scott, Miller, and Griffin, males are more commonly represented.[6]

Kwochka indicates that chronic, relapsing deep pyoderma is more common in short-coated breeds, possibly due to a more intense foreign body reaction to keratin.[8] Certainly, chronic, relapsing pedal pyoderma is more common in short-coated breeds. These data support the hypothesis of secondarily infected follicular retention cysts.

Differential Diagnosis and Diagnosis

Pododemodicosis is the most important differential to rule out for pedal folliculitis and furunculosis. In addition to being a primary differential diagnosis, demodicosis of the feet commonly initiates secondary deep pyoderma. Other diagnostic differentials include secondarily infected foreign body granulomas (foxtails), subcutaneous and deep mycosis, and opportunistic fungal diseases. Severe dermatophytosis and *Pelodera* dermatitis are seen less commonly and can mimic pedal folliculitis and furunculosis.

Diagnosis is accomplished by skin scrapings (to rule in or out underlying demodicosis), microscopic examination of stained smears of exudates (to evaluate for the presence of and identify pathogenic organisms), histopathology, and, possibly, bacterial and fungal cultures. If substantial scar tissue is present, skin scrapings may not be successful in identifying underlying demodicosis. Consequently, skin biopsy may be necessary to rule out pododemodicosis. Demodectic mites may be especially difficult to find by skin scrapings in the Chinese shar-pei.

Ideally, early lesions should be sampled for skin biopsy. Intact pustules, nodules, or hemorrhagic bullae are most likely to yield diagnostic results. The histopathologic lesions seen with pedal folliculitis and furunculosis are similar to those associated with other deep pyodermas.[5]

Once a diagnosis of pedal folliculitis and furunculosis has been established, the clinician must aggressively pursue the identification and management of underlying causes. The presence or absence of initiating pruritus is an important diagnostic clue because pedal pyoderma secondary to allergic disease should be preceded by pruritus.

Therapeutic Overview and Prognosis

Pedal folliculitis and furunculosis is a frustrating disease. Lesions tend to become chronic, and scar tissue impedes drainage and antibiotic penetration. Chronicity also diminishes the likeli-

> **Pedal folliculitis and furunculosis is a frustrating disease. Lesions tend to become chronic, and scar tissue impedes drainage and antibiotic penetration.**

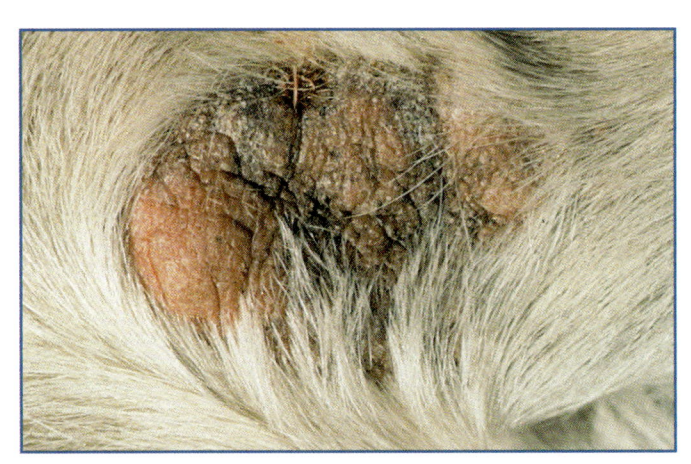

FIGURE 8-15 *Callus pyoderma on the elbow of an adult Labrador retriever. Impacted hair follicles led to deep secondary infection. Bacterial infection is not visually obvious.*

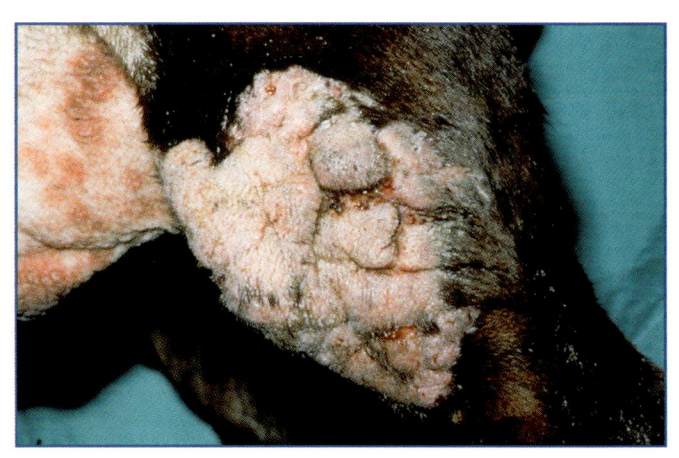

FIGURE 8-16 *Chronic, severe callus pyoderma in a beagle crossbreed with iatrogenic hyperglucocorticoidism and canine atopic dermatitis.*

hood of determining underlying causes. The identification of underlying causes is fundamental to the successful management of this syndrome. Systemic antibiotics are indicated for a minimum of 4 to 6 weeks and at least 2 weeks beyond the resolution of all lesions.

Adjunctive topical therapy is very important in the management of pedal folliculitis and furunculosis. Antibacterial soaks are especially beneficial. Chlorhexidine, povidone-iodine, or boric acid may be added to warm water (see Chapter 10). Daily soaks are advantageous. Antibacterial shampoos can be utilized in a manner similar to that used in the management of other deep pyodermas.

CALLUS PYODERMA (PRESSURE-POINT PYODERMA)

General Considerations

Callus pyoderma develops on calluses located on bony prominences or other pressure points as a sequela to repeated trauma. Calluses form as a normal protective response to repeated pressure trauma. Uninflamed calluses are characterized histologically by dilated, keratin-filled hair follicles. When these abnormal hair follicles rupture due to repeated trauma, hairs are traumatically displaced into the dermis and subcutis. A foreign body response is elicited, and secondary infection ensues, which creates callus pyoderma.[5]

Clinical Findings

Well-demarcated circular or oval lichenified plaques form over bony prominences or other pressure points. Early developing calluses are inflamed, whereas older calluses may be white or grayish due to poorly vascularized excess fibrous connective tissue. Pigmentations vary by breed and chronicity. Alopecia is progressive, and comedones and prominent dilated follicular ostia are common. Multiple hairs may emanate from abnormal, large hair follicles formed as a result of scarring. Although intact furuncles or fistulous tracts may be present, the extent of secondary pyoderma may not be obvious (Figure 8-15). Calluses form most commonly on the elbow, hock, sternum, stifle joint, or lateral digits or over pelvic bony prominences.[5]

Signalment Predilections

Large- or giant-breed dogs are at increased risk. Doberman pinschers, Great Danes, Saint Bernards, Newfoundlands, and Irish wolfhounds frequently develop calluses. Short-legged dogs with poorly protective short hair coats such as smooth-coated dachshunds and basset hounds develop sternal calluses. Although calluses may develop at any age if inciting stimuli are present, untreated calluses enlarge over time (Figure 8-16).

Differential Diagnosis and Diagnosis

Clinical diagnostic differentials are few; calluses are characteristic. Acral lick dermatitis, generic dog food skin disease, and focal actinic comedones share certain clinical features of calluses and callus pyoderma. Acral lick dermatitis and aggregations of actinic comedones are not associated with pressure points. The progression of generic dog food skin disease is different, and, although sites near pressure points are affected, the lesions are clinically dissimilar.

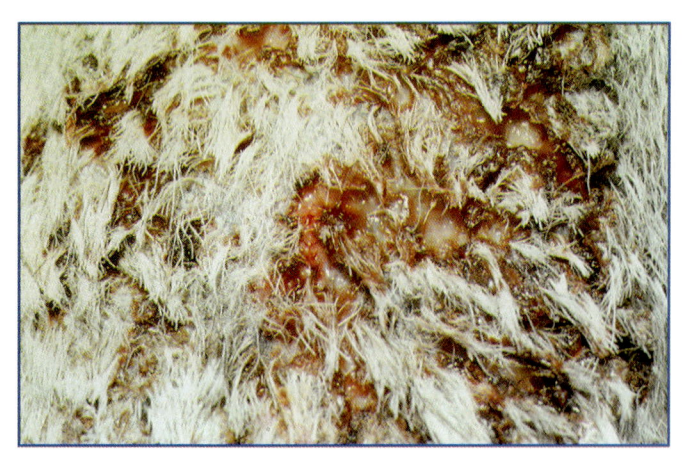

FIGURE 8-17 Lateral thigh region of a dog with German shepherd dog pyoderma. Note the confluent areas of infection and the copious drainage. (Courtesy of Dr. Lynn Schmeitzel, case material, University of California.)

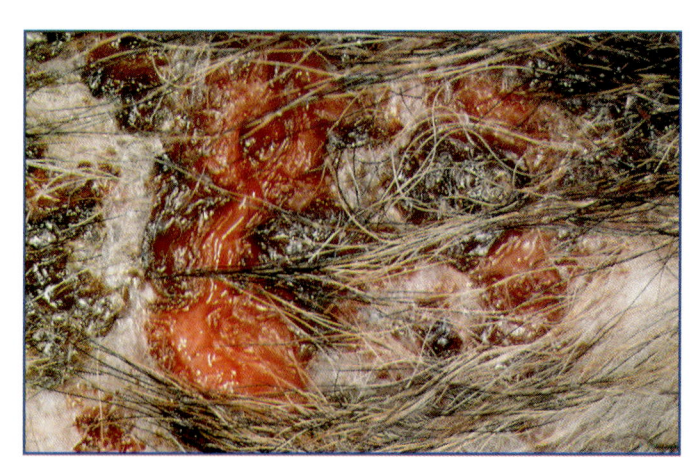

FIGURE 8-18 Close-up of a lesion of German shepherd dog pyoderma. Infected plaques are coalescing. (Courtesy of Dr. Carlo Vitale, case material, University of California.)

Clinical diagnosis usually is sufficient to institute therapy. Skin biopsy is diagnostic, but potential risk must be assessed because healing may be prolonged over bony prominences or pressure points. Histopathology reveals severely acanthotic and hyperplastic epidermis and follicular infundibula. The rupture of dilated, cystic hair follicles provokes severe suppurative and pyogranulomatous inflammation with trichogranulomas.[5]

Therapeutic Overview and Prognosis

Calluses and callus pyoderma are problematic. Behavioral modification directed toward preventing the dog from lying on hard, rough surfaces is integral to treatment. Weight reduction is required if obesity is an additional predisposing factor. Systemic antibiotic therapy should be initiated along with restricting access to hard surfaces. Callus pyoderma requires at least 6 weeks of aggressive antibiotic therapy. Higher antibiotic doses may be necessary because sequestered foci of infection may be shielded by granulomatous inflammation.

Surgical extirpation of a callus may be curative; however, the procedure is fraught with technical difficulties. Dehiscence is a potential complication. Surgical removal may be accomplished more easily with sternal calluses.

GERMAN SHEPHERD DOG PYODERMA
General Considerations

German shepherd folliculitis, furunculosis, and cellulitis (or for simplicity, **German shepherd dog pyoderma**) is an aggressive, deep bacterial infection of the skin of uncertain etiology seen predominantly in German shepherds and related crossbreeds.[13-17] Wisselink and his group have documented a familial predisposition in the German shepherd breed and have hypothesized an autosomal recessive inheritance.[13,14]

Although a defect in cell-mediated immunity has been documented in a small number of dogs, most studies have not been able to elucidate any underlying immunologic abnormality.[14,17,18] Underlying allergic disease or hypothyroidism has been documented in some dogs.[18] Controversy exists with respect to the role of flea allergy dermatitis in this syndrome.[15-18] The author believes that available historical information plus the distribution pattern of German shepherd dog pyoderma suggest that flea allergy dermatitis can be an important trigger in the initiation and recurrence of this syndrome, similar to the original suggestions of Krick and Scott.[15] However, well-defined underlying causes of German shepherd dog pyoderma are not identified in most cases.

Clinical Findings

Erythematous papules, pustules, furuncles, and fistulous tracts develop rapidly, forming confluent plaques of ulcerated and eroded, devitalized skin (Figures 8-17 and 8-18). Adherent crusting is dramatic and, in heavily haired regions, may shield the lesions such that their extent and severity are not recognized by the owner or the veterinarian. Hyperpigmentation is common with chronicity. Pruritus and pain are usually present and may be severe. Peripheral lymphadenopathy is common. Skin lesions are disproportionately severe in comparison to most other pyodermas, with the exception of those seen secondary to generalized demodicosis. Systemic signs may be evident in more severe cases. Severely affected dogs may be anorectic and cachectic. The clinical course of German shepherd dog pyoderma is chronic. Deep folliculitis and furunculosis may eventuate into cellulitis (see below).

The clinical distribution of the syndrome is distinctive. The lateral thighs, rump, dorsal back, and ventral abdomen are commonly the most severely affected sites. The syndrome may generalize, whereby the chest wall and the neck are additional severely affected sites.

Signalment Predilections

As indicated above, this syndrome is seen predominantly in German shepherds and related crossbreeds. However, clinically and histologically similar infection has been occasionally seen in dalmatians and bullterriers. Middle-aged German shepherds may develop the syndrome more frequently.[6]

Differential Diagnosis and Diagnosis

The major clinical differential diagnosis for German shepherd dog pyoderma is deep pyoderma secondary to underlying demodicosis. In addition, subcutaneous and deep mycosis and opportunistic fungal diseases could conceivably mimic this syndrome in German shepherds.

German shepherd dog pyoderma is clinically distinctive due to the character and overwhelming severity of the skin lesions and distribution pattern. Physical examination, evaluation of stained smears from the fistulous tracts, and negative skin scrapings should confirm the presence of deep pyoderma without underlying demodicosis. Skin biopsy should be performed to rule out other possible diseases, confirm the presence of tissue damage severe enough to support the diagnosis, and evaluate for the presence of underlying diseases. Histopathologic findings include severe bacterial deep folliculitis, furunculosis, and cellulitis with severe pyogranulomatous inflammation.[13,15]

Therapeutic Overview and Prognosis

German shepherd dog pyoderma is a severe, frustrating, highly aggressive skin disease. The clinician must evaluate dogs for the presence of underlying triggers or predisposing causes such as immunological incompetence (see Chapter 9), allergic diseases, and hypothyroidism.

Long-term systemic antibiotic therapy must be maintained. In most cases, a minimum of 10 to 12 weeks of therapy is required. Higher antibiotic doses may be beneficial because sequestered foci of infection may impede antibiotic penetration. Caution should be exercised before therapy is withdrawn as relapses may be swift and aggressive. Immunomodulation is controversial but has been beneficial in a limited number of cases.[17]

Initial hospitalization is recommended. Topical therapy is essential to successful management. Although the severity of the disease may be masked by matted debris in a dense hair coat, clipping a "window" so that the owner can visualize the extent and severity of infection is recommended before hospitalization. Whole body clipping is usually required because the dense hair coat may inhibit drainage. For initial therapy, antibacterial shampoos should be used daily, followed by either whirlpools or soaks, as discussed in the section on deep bacterial folliculitis and furunculosis.

Concomitant corticosteroid therapy is absolutely *contraindicated* in the initial management of this syndrome and can lead to catastrophic, fulminating infection. However, in a limited number of cases, corticosteroids at antiinflammatory doses have been successfully used later in the course of the disease (after at least 6 weeks of appropriate systemic antibiotic therapy) to diminish the inappropriate magnitude of inflammation seen in this syndrome.[19] Adjunctive corticosteroid therapy is potentially perilous and is recommended only after consultation with a veterinary dermatologist during hospitalization of the dog.

CELLULITIS
General Considerations

The use of the term *cellulitis* is controversial in veterinary dermatology. By convention, cellulitis has been used to describe a chronic, deep bacterial infection characterized by diffuse, rapidly spreading, suppurative inflammation that is poorly defined and tends to dissect widely along and through tissue planes involving the dermis and subcutaneous tissues[1-3,9] (Figure 8-19). Conversely, cellulitis in humans is an acute

> Higher antibiotic doses may be beneficial in cases of German shepherd dog pyoderma because sequestered foci of infection may impede antibiotic penetration.

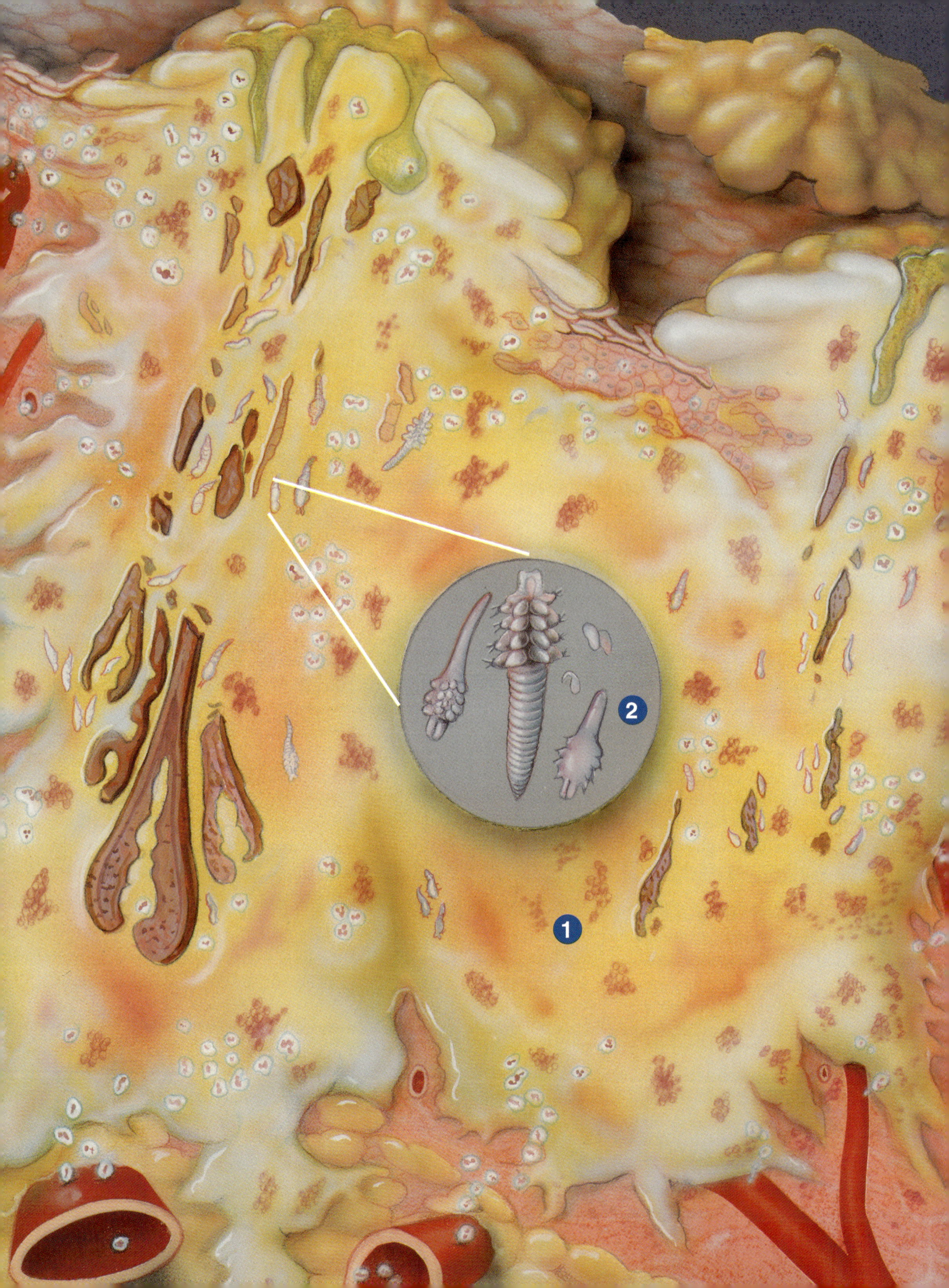
2
1

inflammatory process located predominantly in the deeper subcutaneous tissue that spares the dermis.[20] The term *carbuncle*, used in human medicine, is actually closer to the syndrome known as cellulitis in dogs, although canine lesions are multiple and less discrete then those seen in carbuncles in humans.

Canine cellulitis develops by extension from deep bacterial folliculitis and furunculosis. It occurs most commonly secondary to generalized demodicosis (Figure 8-20). Cellulitis also may be seen secondary to either primary or acquired immunodeficiency. Hypothyroidism, naturally occurring hyperglucocorticoidism, and iatrogenic hyperglucocorticoidism may be underlying causes of canine cellulitis. The deep folliculitis and furunculosis seen predominantly in German shepherds may progress to cellulitis. Any deep pyoderma, especially if managed inappropriately, may potentially develop into cellulitis.

Much of the information discussed in the section on deep bacterial folliculitis and furunculosis also applies to cellulitis. However, cellulitis is a more severe manifestation of bacterial skin disease and may be more frequently life-threatening. The potential for sepsis is always a concern with canine bacterial cellulitis.

Clinical Findings

The lesions of cellulitis tend to be visually more severe than those seen in other deep pyodermas. Boggy edematous plaques with poorly defined borders form, and pus usually oozes from multiple devitalized sites rather than drains from discrete fistulas. Lesions may be exceedingly friable, and the surface may be a discolored grey and appear gelatinous. Simple manipulation during physical examination may severely damage the skin. Site predilections parallel those of the underlying disease (especially demodicosis) or are identical to those seen in other deep pyodermas. Pain or pruritus is commonly present. Lymphadenopathy is usually present and may be regional or generalized.

Signalment Predilections

Cellulitis secondary to generalized demodicosis obviously follows the predilections of the underlying demodicosis. Although various dog breeds have been incriminated as having heritable deficiencies in immune function (e.g., basset hound, collie, Doberman pinscher, Irish setter, bullterrier) an increased frequency of cellulitis has not been noted.

Differential Diagnosis and Diagnosis

Cellulitis should be differentiated from other less severe forms of pyoderma. Smears of pus should be stained and evaluated for the presence of cocci and other bacteria. Skin biopsy should be performed to rule out other diseases, confirm the presence of tissue damage severe enough to support the diagnosis of cellulitis, and evaluate for the presence of underlying diseases. Histopathologic findings include severe pyogranulomatous inflammation involving hair follicles, the interfollicular dermis, and the underlying subcutis.

The presence or absence of underlying demodicosis must be determined by multiple, deep skin scrapings. If demodicosis is not present, the clinician must aggressively pursue the identification of other factors leading to immunosuppression.

Other nonbacterial skin diseases that can clinically mimic bacterial cellulitis

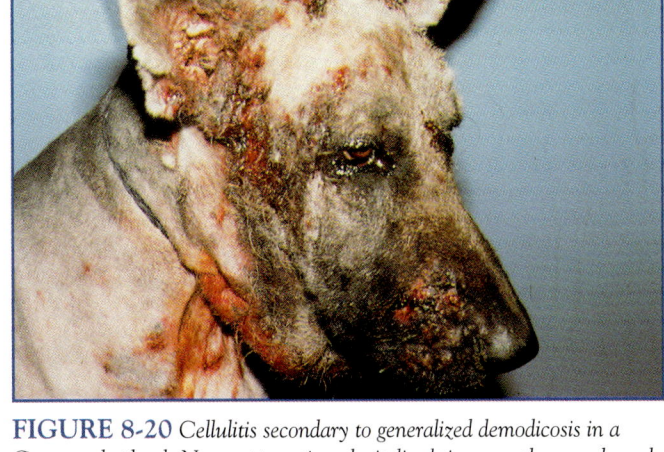

FIGURE 8-20 *Cellulitis secondary to generalized demodicosis in a German shepherd. Note suppurative, devitalized tissue on the muzzle and below the ear. (Courtesy of Dr. Mitchell Song, case material, University of California.)*

> In cases of cellulitis, smears of pus should be stained and evaluated for the presence of cocci and other bacteria.

FIGURE 8-19 *Cellulitis secondary to generalized demodicosis. (1) Infection is poorly defined and encompasses the dermis and underlying subcutaneous tissues. (2) Demodectic mites and mite fragments free from a hair follicle within the region of cellulitis.*

include juvenile sterile granulomatous dermatitis and lymphadenitis (juvenile cellulitis), subcutaneous and deep mycosis, sterile granuloma/pyogranuloma, and idiopathic sterile liquefying panniculitis.

Therapeutic Overview and Prognosis

Cellulitis is always a therapeutic challenge. Management is similar to that of other severe deep pyodermas. However, underlying sepsis and systemic signs are more likely. If the cellulitis is secondary to demodicosis or another identified immunosuppressive disease, the primary underlying disease must be managed appropriately. Dogs with cellulitis secondary to primary or acquired immunodeficiency not associated with an identifiable underlying disease have a guarded prognosis and require long-term antibacterial therapy. Immunomodulatory therapy may be attempted (see Chapter 10).

---

[a]Bactoderm®, Pfizer Animal Health.

REFERENCES

1. Ihrke PJ: An overview of bacterial skin disease in the dog. *Br Vet J* 433:112–118, 1987.
2. White SD, Ihrke PJ: Pyoderma, in Nesbitt GH (ed): *Dermatology—Contemporary Issues in Small Animal Practice*. New York, Churchill Livingstone, 1987, pp 95–121.
3. Ihrke PJ: Bacterial infections of the skin, in Greene CE (ed): *Infectious Diseases of the Dog and Cat*. Philadelphia, WB Saunders, 1990, pp 72–79.
4. Carlotti D, Fourrier P, Magnol J-P: Les pyodermites profondes. *Prat Med Chirurg Anim Compag* 23:487–497, 1988.
5. Gross TL, Ihrke PJ, Walder EJ: *Veterinary Dermatopathology: A Macroscopic and Microscopic Evaluation of Canine and Feline Skin Disease*. St. Louis, Mosby–Year Book, 1992, pp 10–14, 238–240, 252–255.
6. Scott DW, Miller WH, Griffin CE: *Muller & Kirk's Small Animal Dermatology*, ed 5. Philadelphia, WB Saunders, 1995, pp 279–328.
7. Gross TL: Canine eosinophilic furunculosis of the face, in Ihrke PJ, Mason IS, White SD (eds): *Advances in Veterinary Dermatology*, vol 2. Oxford, Pergamon Press, 1992, pp 239–246.
8. Kwochka KW: Recurrent pyoderma, in Griffin CE, Kwochka KW, Macdonald JM (eds): *Current Veterinary Dermatology*. St. Louis, Mosby–Year Book, 1993, pp 3–21.
9. Muller GH, Kirk RW, Scott DW: *Small Animal Dermatology*, ed 4. Philadelphia, WB Saunders, 1989, pp 739–740.
10. Reinke SI, Stannard AA, Ihrke PJ, et al: Histopathologic features of pyotraumatic dermatitis. *JAVMA* 190:57–60, 1987.
11. White SD: Pododermatitis. *Vet Dermatol* 1(1):1–18, 1989.
12. Gross TL: Unpublished data, 1993.
13. Wisselink MA, Willemse A, Koeman JP: Deep pyoderma in the German shepherd dog. *JAAHA* 21:773–776, 1985.
14. Wisselink MA, Bernadina WE, Willemse A, Noordzij A: Immunologic aspects of German shepherd dog pyoderma (GSP). *Vet Immunol Immunopathol* 19:67–77, 1988.
15. Krick SA, Scott DW: Bacterial folliculitis, furunculosis and cellulitis in the German shepherd dog: A retrospective analysis of 17 cases. *JAAHA* 25:23–30, 1989.
16. Buerger RG: Staphylococci and German shepherd pyoderma, in Kirk RW (ed): *Current Veterinary Therapy X*. Philadelphia, WB Saunders, 1989, pp 609–614.
17. Miller WH Jr: Deep pyoderma in two German shepherd dogs associated with a cell-mediated immunodeficiency. *JAAHA* 27:513–517, 1991.
18. Rosser EJ Jr: German shepherd pyoderma: A prospective study of 12 dogs. Proceedings of the American Academy/College of Veterinary Dermatology, 9:40–42, 1993.
19. Olivry T, Ihrke PJ: Unpublished data, 1993.
20. Weinberg AN, Swartz MN: Bacterial diseases with cutaneous involvement. in Fitzpatrick TB, Eisen AZ, Wolff K, et al (eds): *Dermatology in General Medicine*, ed 4. New York, McGraw-Hill, 1993, pp 2297–2309.

Chapter 9

Diagnostic Procedures Useful in Canine Pyoderma

GENERAL CONSIDERATIONS

Many diagnostic procedures may be beneficial in diagnosing bacterial infections of the skin and documenting underlying diseases or factors leading to initiation or recurrence. However, certain procedures are more likely to efficiently and economically provide useful diagnostic information. Skin scrapings, cytologic examination, and skin biopsy are the most consistently useful diagnostic procedures in the evaluation of suspected canine pyoderma.[1,2] Bacterial culture, identification, and antibiotic sensitivity testing frequently are overused in cases of superficial pyoderma and even in deep pyoderma. Cytologic examination of material harvested by either smears of pustular contents or draining fistulous tracts commonly yields as much or more useful information than bacterial cultures and is more cost effective and rapid.[1-3] Skin scrapings should be performed in all suspected or documented cases of canine pyoderma because demodicosis can initiate lesions identical to those seen with uncomplicated pyoderma. Skin biopsy often is neglected as a valuable tool in the diagnosis of canine pyoderma.

Results obtained from laboratory evaluation for immunocompetency in cases of canine pyoderma are frequently disappointing. However, under certain circumstances, an evaluation for immunologic competency is indicated.[1,4]

SKIN SCRAPINGS

Skin scrapings for potential underlying demodicosis are important in the evaluation of any dog with suspected or proven pyoderma. Any superficial or deep pyoderma with a follicular orientation should have multiple skin scrapings performed to rule out underlying demodicosis.[1-3] Skin scrapings are most likely to yield demodectic mites in lip-fold intertrigo, superficial folliculitis, deep folliculitis and furunculosis, and cellulitis.[5]

Because intense follicular colonization by demodectic mites tends to favor deep, perforating bacterial follicular disease, deep pyoderma is more likely to be seen secondary to demodicosis. In deep pyoderma, the syndromes with the potential of underlying demodicosis that should be most aggressively pursued include muzzle folliculitis and furunculosis (canine acne), pedal folliculitis and furunculosis, German shepherd dog pyoderma, and cellulitis. It is important to remember that underlying demodicosis cannot be unequivocally ruled out by skin scrapings. Demodicosis has been documented by skin biopsy following negative skin scrapings in the Chinese shar-pei and in various breeds that have pedal folliculitis and furunculosis with excessive scar tissue and chronic inflammation.

Deep skin scraping for the identification of demodectic mites may be performed either with a scalpel blade or a skin-scraping spatula.[6-8] Skin-scraping spatulas have the advantage of diminished chance of accidental laceration.[7] Hair should always be clipped from the affected area before scraping. Close but gentle clipping, utilizing an electric clipper with a #40 blade, greatly increases the likelihood of harvesting demodectic mites in skin scrapings. Although alopecia is not always a feature of generalized demodicosis in dogs with long anagen hair cycles, underlying demodicosis must always be suspected in any cases of recurrent deep pyoderma, especially if lesions occur at unusual sites[5] (see Chapter 13).

Scrapings are best accomplished with either a #10 or #15 scalpel blade or a special-purpose skin-scraping spatula. The author recommends holding the scalpel blade, without an attached handle, between the thumb and second finger, using the first finger to guard against laceration. The blade is moistened with a medium-grade mineral oil, and the scraping is performed in the direction of hair growth with the blade held perpendicular to the skin surface. The acquired specimen is spread evenly on a microscope slide, covered with a coverslip, and examined under a microscope, utilizing low levels of light with maximum contrast (condenser down); a scanning and low-powered objective is used. Other scraping media such as potassium hydroxide are not recommended because they kill the harvested mites. Live mites are identified more readily, and the preparations may be used to determine live:dead mite ratios that can be important prognosticators in managing generalized demodicosis.

CYTOLOGIC EXAMINATION

Cytologic examination is one of the easiest, most cost-effective, and potentially most beneficial diagnostic tests for the documentation of bacterial involvement in canine skin disease[1,3,7,8] (Table 9-1). Depending on the lesion, either a smear of pustular contents or fine-needle aspiration can be performed. Smears of pustular contents are recommended for intact pustules and draining fistulous tracts. If skin biopsy is performed on deep lesions for histopathology, the biopsy specimen can be blotted gently on a slide before it is placed in formalin. In addition, surface lesions, including pyotraumatic dermatitis, intertrigo, and mucocutaneous pyoderma, should be smeared to verify the presence of bacteria and rule out the presence of *Malassezia* organisms.

Intact pustules can be opened with a 25- or 26-gauge hypodermic needle. The pustular contents can be directly transferred with the needle and smeared on a microscope slide. A cotton-tipped swab may be used to touch the material draining from a fistulous tract and transfer it to a microscope slide. Alternatively and rarely, if owners will not support skin biopsy, cavitated nodules, pustules, vesicles, or bullae may be aspirated with a 22-gauge needle attached to a 3-ml syringe.

Specimens are air dried and stained using either a modified Romanovsky-type Wright's stain[a] or new methylene blue. The modified Wright's stain is recommended for cytologic examination to evaluate for the presence of organisms and for the identification of inflammatory cells.

The finding of cocci is highly suggestive of pyoderma caused by *Staphylococcus intermedius*. The absence of bacteria within the contents of a pustule, vesicle, or bullae usually indicates that the lesions are not bacterial in origin. The finding of rod-shaped bacteria accompanying cocci indicates the presence of mixed infection. The author agrees with the recently published clinical observations of Scott, Miller, and Griffin, indicating that fewer bacteria (with the majority located inside inflammatory cells) are seen in specimens from deep pyoderma and that the presence of abnormally large numbers of cocci within pustules indicates the likelihood of underlying endogenous or iatrogenic hyperglucocorticoidism.[3] Similar findings have been noted in dogs receiving immunosuppressive cytotoxic therapy for cancer or autoimmune diseases.

The presence of neutrophils with degenerative or cytologic changes supports the diagnosis of pyoderma, especially if some cocci are located intracellularly. The additional presence of macrophages or giant cells suggests that the infection is deeper and chronic.

SKIN BIOPSY

Skin biopsy is a valuable tool for diagnosing and evaluating cases of canine pyoderma.[1-3,5] The more often skin diseases are biopsied, the more commonly pyoderma is diagnosed, even when bacterial skin disease is not initially suspected.[1] Adhering to certain basic principles will maximize the benefits derived from taking a skin biopsy. The indications, timing, lesion selection, biopsy method selection, biopsy technique, preparation for submission, and selection of a pathologist are all critical factors in maximizing the benefits of skin biopsy.[5,9]

TABLE 9-1
HOW TO PERFORM CYTOLOGIC EXAMINATION

PROCEDURE

Intact Pustules
- Open with a 25- or 26-gauge needle. Transfer contents with the needle and smear on a slide.

Draining Fistulous Tracts
- Use a cotton-tipped swab and transfer contents by rolling onto a slide.

STAINING
- Stain dried specimens with a modified Romanovsky-type Wright's stain or new methylene blue.

Indications

The primary reason for performing a skin biopsy is the rapid establishment of a definitive diagnosis. Additional benefits include ruling out other potentially serious diseases and identifying unexpected underlying diseases. Neoplasia may visually resemble certain pyodermas. For example, sweat gland adenocarcinomas may clinically mimic pyotraumatic dermatitis (see Chapter 6). Skin biopsy of chronic pedal folliculitis and furunculosis may unexpectedly identify demodectic mites not found on skin scrapings (see Chapter 8 and above). After a diagnosis has been established, repeat skin biopsy can be used to assay response to therapy and predict prognosis. Prognostic skin biopsy is underutilized in veterinary medicine for financial reasons.

Timing and Lesion Selection

Skin biopsy should be performed as soon as possible in the course of disease to maximize the likelihood of reaching a definitive diagnosis. Early primary lesions more frequently yield diagnostic information. Intact pustules, nodules, and hemorrhagic bullae are more likely to yield useful information than secondary crusted papules, ulcers, or erosions.

Obtaining multiple biopsy specimens increases the likelihood of obtaining a diagnosis. Lesions that are most representative of the disease process should be selected for skin biopsy. If the skin lesions vary considerably in character, multiple lesions that are different in appearance should be sampled because they may represent different stages in the evolution of the disease. Multiple biopsies also are important when clinical lesions are subtle. Most diagnostic pathology laboratories will process two or three specimens representing the same disease process for the same fee as long as the specimens fit into a single processing cassette.[5]

Biopsy Method Selection

Wedge biopsy or punch biopsy procedures may be used for sampling suspected bacterial infections. Each procedure has advantages and disadvantages. The advantages of wedge biopsy include obtaining a larger specimen, causing less trauma to fragile lesions, and providing ease of specimen orientation in the laboratory. Advantages of punch biopsy include the speed of the procedure and greater client acceptance. In addition, punch biopsy results in a smaller surgical wound than that caused by wedge biopsy.

Elliptical wedge biopsy specimens obtained with a scalpel can be oriented easily by the laboratory technician to ensure better sectioning. Fragile lesions such as large pustules, vesicopustules, or hemorrhagic bullae are less likely to be damaged by wedge biopsy. If the disease is suspected to involve the panniculus, wedge biopsy is necessary because subcutaneous tissue is not obtained reliably in most punch biopsy specimens. However, wedge biopsy requires more time and multiple sutures and dogs may require general anesthesia. Because of these negative features, wedge biopsy is employed less frequently than punch biopsy.

Punch biopsy has the substantial advantages of ease of specimen procurement by using local anesthesia, and the procedure results in a minimal surgical wound. Consequently, punch biopsy is less expensive, and many dog owners are more likely to allow the procedure to be performed on their dogs because of these advantages. The speed of punch biopsies also facilitates taking multiple specimens, optimizing the diagnostic benefit of the procedure. The disadvantages of punch biopsy include predetermined smaller sample size and the shearing trauma to fragile lesions created by rotating a biopsy punch.

Skin Biopsy Technique

Sampling technique varies between wedge and punch biopsy. An elliptical wedge biopsy can include a transitional zone and a small amount of normal tissue at one pole of the wedge since the technician can easily orient the tissue and, by convention, transects the specimen through its long axis. Conversely, punch biopsy specimens should only include abnormal tissue. If normal tissue is included using this procedure, routine processing and embedment of one half of the specimen may eliminate most or all of the lesional tissue.

> Cytologic examination is one of the easiest, most cost-effective, and potentially most beneficial diagnostic tests for the documentation of bacterial involvement in canine skin disease.

Wedge biopsy specimens must not exceed 2 cm in width or length because larger specimens may not fix adequately in formalin. Disposable skin biopsy punches of 4, 6, and 8 mm in diameter are used most commonly. Punches of 6 or 8 mm are recommended for the biopsy of most pyodermas. Biopsy punches of 4 mm are reserved for difficult areas such as the muzzle, lips, and periorbital sites, because smaller biopsy specimens are more likely to exhibit procurement artifact and are less likely to yield a diagnosis.

A separate cold sterilization tray containing the required instruments is recommended to expedite the skin biopsy procedure, which will be performed more often if the necessary instrumentation is available. Proper handling of fragile tissue is imperative and is facilitated by the use of small surgical instruments designed for use in ophthalmology. Curved iris scissors and fine-eye forceps should be included. Small curved hemostats, a small needle holder, suture scissors, and a small scalpel handle also are recommended. Disposable 8, 6, and 4 mm punches may be placed on the cold sterilization tray after initial use and reused two or three times.

Local anesthesia and physical restraint are sufficient for most procedures. Tranquilization or general anesthesia may be indicated in a fractious dog or when lesions are localized to the muzzle or periorbital, digital, or interdigital regions. Skin biopsy sites are clipped carefully to remove hair without creating inflammation and should *not* be cleansed or prepared in any way because surface material is an important part of the specimen.

An indelible marker is used to indicate the site of biopsy to prevent inadvertent sampling of nonblocked areas. Four dots are placed equidistant from the site. Lidocaine (2%) is used routinely for local anesthesia. If the barrel of the syringe is rinsed with epinephrine before withdrawing the lidocaine, hemostasis will be facilitated and the spread of the local anesthetic will be restricted. One milliliter of lidocaine is sufficient for each site. The lidocaine is introduced sublesionally into the subcutaneous tissue directly under the lesion using a 25-gauge needle. Blockage with minimal patient discomfort is achieved by gently repositioning the needle without removing it from the initial site and depositing the anesthetic in a fanlike pattern. Because sensory nerves radiate from the spinal column, the side of the biopsy site closest to the spine is recommended so that needle repositioning will not cause additional patient discomfort. Skin biopsy is performed between 5 and 8 minutes after the injection of local anesthetic.

If the infection is suspected of invading subcutaneous fat (e.g., cellulitis and German shepherd dog pyoderma), ring block, regional anesthesia, or general anesthesia should be performed to allow the subcutaneous part of the lesion to be sampled without artifact created from subcutaneous lidocaine usage.

The disposable biopsy punch is rotated gently in one direction until the blade has entered the subcutaneous tissue. (The punch is rotated in one direction only because back-and-forth rotation may increase the likelihood of specimen damage from shearing forces). The clinician should note an easing of pressure when the punch has successfully entered the subcutaneous tissue.

The biopsy specimen is removed gently with a pair of fine-eye forceps and curved iris scissors. Because unfixed tissue is fragile, the specimen should be grasped gently only by hair stubble, subcutaneous fat, or the edge of the dermal–epidermal junction. Artifacts rendering the specimen useless are readily introduced by excessive manipulation. Blood can be blotted by gently rolling the specimen on absorbent paper toweling. A small piece of a wooden tongue depressor or cardboard can be used as a splint to preserve proper anatomic orientation and prevent distortion of the specimen during fixation. The specimen should be placed on the splint with the subcutaneous side down. The splint is floated or emersed, specimen side down, in the fixative. The biopsy specimen should be placed in the fixative as soon as possible because artifactual changes can occur within 1 minute after sample procurement.

Suturing of the biopsy site is required with wedge biopsy and larger punch biopsies. Punch sites of 4 mm do not require suturing. Larger (6 or 8 mm) punch biopsy sites

> Skin biopsy may provide rapid establishment of a definitive diagnosis and help to rule out other potentially serious diseases and identify unexpected underlying diseases.

require either a purse-string suture or several simple interrupted sutures.

Neutral phosphate-buffered formalin (10%) is the fixative recommended for routine histopathologic evaluation. The volume of fixative should be at least 10 times the volume of the specimen for proper fixation. Fixation requires 12 hours before processing for histopathology. Formalin freezes at −11°C (12.2°F). Specimens should be maintained at room temperature for 6 hours before exposure to extreme cold to prevent them from freezing.

Preparation for Submission

Ideally, specimens should be submitted to a veterinary pathologist specializing in dermatopathology. If a dermatopathologist is not available, a general veterinary pathologist with an interest in dermatology should be selected. It is essential that signalment information (i.e., breed, age, and sex) and a brief description of the clinical findings are included with the biopsy specimen. Clinical descriptions are, in fact, the "gross pathology" and are essential in establishing a diagnosis.[5]

BACTERIAL CULTURE, IDENTIFICATION, AND ANTIBIOTIC SENSITIVITY

Although potentially useful, bacterial culture, identification, and antibiotic sensitivity testing frequently are overused in the evaluation and management of canine pyoderma. These modalities may be indicated in mixed infections (as determined by cytologic evaluation) and in any cases of pyoderma where appropriate empiric antibiotic therapy has not been efficacious.[1]

In-house bacterial culture should not be performed in veterinary hospitals. Specimens should be sent to a veterinary diagnostic laboratory with a microbiologist familiar with veterinary pathogens and saprophytes.[7]

Lesion selection and careful specimen handling are critical to achieving authoritative, reproducible results. In general, bacterial cultures should not be performed on open lesions. Cultures of intact pustules, furuncles, or nodules are more likely to yield useful information, whereas open lesions simply document the organisms (pathogens and contaminants) that may live on an ideal culture medium. Draining fistulous tracts may be cultured if closed lesions are unavailable for culture in cases of deep pyoderma. However, care must be taken to harvest pus from a fistula after surface debris has been cleansed away.

The area to be cultured should be clipped if hair near the pustule is likely to contaminate the specimen during collection. Controversy exists as to the advisability of cleansing the surface before sampling a closed pustule.[1–3,7,8] The author routinely blots the collection site with alcohol and allows it to dry before culturing. Others recommend no cleansing whatsoever.[7]

Culturing of intact pustules is accomplished by pricking the pustule with a 22- to 26-gauge needle and transferring the contents to a sterile aerobic culturette swab with an integral ampule of liquid transport medium. The pus attached to the needle must be transferred to the culturette swab well away from the dog so that surrounding hairs do not contaminate the specimen.

Various methods may be employed in the culture of deep pyodermas. If intact fluid-filled furuncles are present, they may be sampled in a similar manner to that of intact superficial pustules. If intact, noncontaminated lesions are not present, the clinician can culture a draining fistulous tract by cleansing the surface and extruding pus from the fistula that has not been contaminated on the surface. Alternatively, a skin biopsy can be taken under sterile conditions and the specimen transferred to a sterile transport container. Communication with the microbiologist is recommended so that the specimen is sent according to their guidelines. The reader is referred to a recent publication by Moriello for additional information.[7]

EVALUATION FOR IMMUNOCOMPETENCY

Laboratory results obtained for the evaluation of immunocompetence in cases of canine pyoderma frequently are disappointing. According to a recent review by DeBoer, "With our current state of knowledge, the advisability or cost-effectiveness of an 'immunological

> When performing bacterial cultures, lesion selection and careful specimen handling are critical to achieving authoritative, reproducible results.

work-up' is questionable on a number of grounds."[4] This is due to both a lack of cases where immunodeficiency has been successfully documented, coupled with the lack of ability to meaningfully assess the protean facets of immune competence referable to bacterial infection in the dog. In addition, many tests are not available to practicing veterinarians or, if available, are prohibitively expensive.[4] A further detractor to testing is our lack of ability to correct documented defects.

Serum immunoglobulin quantitation, complete blood count, serum electrophoresis, lymphocyte blastogenesis assays, and neutrophil function tests all have been suggested as parameters to evaluate immunocompetence in the dog.[1-4,10,11]

Serum immunoglobulin quantitations of immunoglobulin G, immunoglobulin M, and immunoglobulin A can be performed by radial immunodiffusion as well as by other methods. Results may vary substantially from laboratory to laboratory, and comparisons of values between different laboratories can be misleading.[4] Most dogs with pyoderma do not exhibit gross deficiencies in immunoglobulin production.

It also has been suggested that gross information may be derived from a complete blood count and serum electrophoresis. Theoretically, an absolute neutrophilia with a lymphocyte count of at least 1000 cells/µl to 1500 cells/µl of blood should be seen in immunologically normal dogs adequately responding to ongoing or recurrent pyoderma.[1,10] The complete blood count should be repeated if low lymphocyte counts are noted in one sample. Repeatable lymphopenia might indicate lymphocyte dysfunction.[4] A broad-based elevation in the serum electrophoretic pattern in the β and γ range should also be seen in normal dogs responding to bacterial infection.[1,10]

In vitro lymphocyte blastogenesis assays are available principally as research tools. Practicality is limited by extensive equipment requirements and technical difficulties as well as the additional problem that blood samples for this assay must be processed within 2 hours of collection. Neutrophil function tests include phagocytic and bactericidal assays such as the nitroblue tetrazolium reduction assay. Little data referable to clinical significance are available.[4]

> Theoretically, an absolute neutrophilia with a lymphocyte count of at least 1000 cells/µl to 1500 cells/µl of blood should be seen in immunologically normal dogs adequately responding to ongoing or recurrent pyoderma.

---

[a]Diff-Quik®, American Scientific Products.

REFERENCES

1. Ihrke PJ: Bacterial infections of the skin, in Greene CE (ed): *Infectious Diseases of the Dog and Cat.* Philadelphia, WB Saunders, 1990, pp 72–79.
2. Ihrke PJ: Antibacterial therapy in dermatology, in Kirk RW, Bonagura JD (eds): *Current Veterinary Therapy IX.* Philadelphia, WB Saunders, 1986, pp 566–571.
3. Scott DW, Miller WH, Griffin CE: *Muller & Kirk's Small Animal Dermatology,* ed 5. Philadelphia, WB Saunders, 1995, pp 55–173.
4. DeBoer DJ: Management of chronic and recurrent pyoderma in the dog, in Kirk RW, Bonagura JD (eds): *Current Veterinary Therapy IX.* Philadelphia, WB Saunders, 1995, pp 611–617.
5. Gross TL, Ihrke PJ, Walder EJ: *Veterinary Dermatopathology: A Macroscopic and Microscopic Evaluation of Canine and Feline Skin Disease.* St. Louis Mosby–Year Book, 1992, pp 1–326.
6. Ihrke PJ: Skin scrapings in the diagnosis of ectoparasitic skin diseases. *Compend Contin Educ Anim Health Tech II* 1:5–11, 1981.
7. Moriello K: Diagnostic testing, in Moriello KA, Mason IS (eds): *Handbook of Small Animal Dermatology.* Oxford, Pergamon, 1995, pp 19–44.
8. Littlewood J: Investigative and laboratory techniques, in Locke PH, Harvey RG, Mason IS (eds): *Manual of Small Animal Dermatology.* Gloucestershire, BSAVA, 1993, pp 33–44.
9. Ihrke PJ, Gross TL: The skin biopsy: Maximizing benefit. Scientific Proceedings, AAHA 55th Annual Meeting, 1988, pp 299–301.
10. Halliwell REW, Gorman NT: *Veterinary Clinical Immunology.* Philadelphia, WB Saunders, 1989, pp 450–466.
11. Ihrke PJ: An overview of bacterial skin disease in the dog. *Br Vet J* 433:112–118, 1987.

Chapter 10

Overview of the Management of Canine Pyoderma

GENERAL CONSIDERATIONS

Appropriate management of most cases of superficial and deep canine pyoderma requires the use of systemic antibiotics, usually in conjunction with adjunctive topical shampoo therapy.[1-11] Topical antibacterial therapy commonly is used as an adjunct to systemic antibiotics because it may offer enhanced speed of recovery and improve general patient well-being. Antibacterial shampoos also may be used prophylactically to prevent or postpone recurrent infection. Immunomodulatory therapy, although rarely implemented, is used most commonly in an attempt to prevent or diminish the frequency of recurrent infections.[7,9-11] Extended regimens of systemic antibiotics commonly are used as a last resort in the management of chronic, recurrent pyoderma (see Chapter 13).

SYSTEMIC ANTIBIOTIC THERAPY

The basic principles of successful systemic antibiotic therapy for the management of canine pyoderma include choice of the proper antibiotic, establishment of an effective dosage, and long enough maintenance of therapy to ensure cure rather than simply transient remission[2,12] (Table 10-1).

Antibiotics can either be selected empirically or based on the results of bacterial culture, identification, and sensitivity testing. An antibiotic chosen empirically should have a known spectrum of activity against *Staphylococcus intermedius*, the most common canine cutaneous pathogen (Table 10-2). Ideally, the antibiotic should not be inactivated by β-lactamases, although many β-lactamase–resistant antibiotics are more expensive.

Cytology from a pustule or fistulous tract may be performed to verify the suspicion that infection is caused by gram-positive cocci. Ideally, the chosen antibiotic should have a narrow spectrum of activity, minimal side effects, and a reasonable cost as well as being an effective agent in the management of canine pyoderma based on previous use. A second culture should be considered if *S. intermedius* has not been isolated as the primary pathogen (see Chapter 9). If a single, oral antibiotic will not cover multiple isolates, an appropriate antibiotic that is effective against the isolated *S. intermedius* should be chosen initially because this organism creates a tissue milieu favorable to the replication of other secondary bacterial invaders.

Perfusion of skin is less than ideal for establishing adequate dosages of antibiotics, in comparison to other body tissues. According to Ayliffe,[13] only 4% of cardiac output reaches the skin in contrast to 33% of cardiac output reaching muscles. Tissue levels of penicillin antibiotics reached 60% of serum levels in the subcutis and only 40% of serum levels at the dermal–epidermal junction.[11,13] Sequestered foci of infection, foreign body granulomatous response, and antibiotic inactivation by inflammatory products further compromise effective antibiotic dosing in dogs with deep pyoderma (see Chapter 11).

TABLE 10-1
BASIC PRINCIPLES OF SUCCESSFUL SYSTEMIC ANTIBIOTIC THERAPY

- Choice of the proper antibiotic
- Establishment of an effective dosage
- Long enough maintenance of therapy to ensure cure rather than simply transient remission[2,12]

TABLE 10-2
ORAL ANTIBIOTICS USEFUL IN DERMATOLOGY

Drug Name and Dosage	Advantages	Disadvantages	Assessment
Erythromycin (10–15 mg/kg q8h)	Inexpensive; narrow spectrum	Cross-resistance with lincomycin; vomiting and diarrhea common; given three times daily	Good first empiric choice
Lincomycin (22 mg/kg q12h)	Given twice daily; narrow spectrum	Cross-resistance with erythromycin; relatively expensive	Good first empiric choice, especially if q12h drug is needed
Ormetoprim-sulfadimethoxine (27.5 mg/kg q24h)	Given once daily; broad spectrum	Relatively expensive; side effects?	Good first empiric choice, especially if q24h drug is needed
Cephalexin, cefadroxil (22 mg/kg q12h)	Given twice daily; broad spectrum; resistance rare; good tissue penetration	Cefadroxil is expensive	Excellent choices for refractory/recurrent deep pyoderma; q12h drugs
Enrofloxacin (5 mg/kg q24h)	Given once daily; broad spectrum; rapidly absorbed; excellent tissue penetration	Expensive; contraindicated in growing dogs	Excellent choice for refractory/recurrent deep pyoderma; q24h drug
Oxacillin (22 mg/kg q8h)	Narrow spectrum; resistance and side effects rare	Expensive; given three times daily; food interferes with absorption; given 1 hour before feeding	Good choice for refractory/recurrent deep pyoderma
Amoxicillin-clavulanate (12.5–20 mg/kg q12h or q8h!)	Broad spectrum; side effects rare	Expensive; moisture sensitive; in vivo effect not as good as would be predicted?	Efficacy does not warrant expense?; used in cases of deep pyoderma
Trimethoprim-sulfonamides (22 mg/kg q12h)	Inexpensive; given twice daily; broad spectrum	Side effects: keratoconjunctivitis sicca, severe cutaneous drug reactions, hepatic necrosis	Good empiric choice?; concern for drug reactions

The establishment of appropriate antibiotic dosages is controversial in veterinary dermatology. Little work has been done to evaluate optimum, required antibiotic levels for the management of canine pyoderma. Consequently, many recommended antibiotic dosages are empiric, although they are based on results obtained from widespread clinical use. All dogs should be weighed. Dosages used should be as close to established recommendations as possible but should not be less than recommended. Underdosing is likely to lead to diminished efficacy, whereas overdosing may increase the likelihood of adverse reactions with some antibiotics. Underdosing is a more common error in larger dogs; overdosing is more frequent in very small dogs.

Fortunately, many oral antibiotics apparently can be given at higher-than-recommended dosages with reasonable safety. Mason recently stated that "in general, doses of antimicrobial agents are doubled for skin infections so that effective tissue concentrations are more likely to be achieved."[8] Although there is not general acceptance of this view, it illustrates the willingness of dermatologists to increase dosages in patients with skin infections. Increased frequency of vomition is seen with erythromycin and occasionally with other antibiotics, if dosages are increased beyond recommended levels. Dosages of trimethoprim-potentiated sulfonamides above manufacturers' recommendations should be avoided because sulfonamide cystic urolithiasis may occur rapidly in susceptible dogs.[14]

Higher-than-established antibiotic dosages may be necessary in dogs with deep pyoderma, as sequestered foci of infection may be shielded by granulomatous inflammation (see Chapters 8 and 11). While treating deep pyoderma with excessive scarring and sequestered infection, the author has successfully used generic cephalexin and enrofloxacin at dosages ranging from two to four times those normally recommended. Adverse side effects were uncommon and apparently no more frequent than those usually seen with these two antibiotics.

Antibiotic therapy must be maintained until complete elimination of bacterial infection rather than simply transient remission is achieved. This usually necessitates maintaining appropriate levels of antibiotic therapy for at least 1 week beyond clinical cure for superficial pyoderma and a minimum of at least 2 weeks beyond clinical cure in all cases of deep pyoderma because nonvisible sequestered foci of infection often remain after most lesions have cleared. It should be emphasized that surface lesions commonly heal before deeper lesions have resolved in cases of canine deep pyoderma.

Antibiotics are rarely used in veterinary dermatology in accordance with manufacturers' recommendations of total duration of therapy. The suggested maximum durations of therapy listed by most manufacturers fall far short of the time span actually required to ensure cure for most types of canine pyoderma.[15-17]

An in-depth discussion of the clinical pharmacology and mechanisms of action of each antibiotic mentioned is beyond the scope of this manual. Details are given where particular attributes of an antibiotic may be specifically beneficial for the management of pyoderma. The reader is referred to standard veterinary textbooks for more basic information.[18-20]

Culture and Sensitivity Studies

Multiple studies have documented sensitivity and resistance patterns of *S. intermedius* isolated from canine infections worldwide.[21-31] Additional data are available, and sensitivity and resistance patterns also are discussed in various clinical trials.[15-17,32-38]

Penicillin, ampicillin, amoxicillin, tetracycline, and nonpotentiated sulfonamides traditionally have been regarded as poor choices for the management of canine staphylococcal pyoderma in the United States and Canada, based on sensitivity and resistance patterns and subjective clinical experience.[1-4,11,12] One proceedings, published 15 years ago, indicated that ampicillin and amoxicillin were much more efficacious for the management of canine pyoderma in England than in North America, but few details were given.[23] More recent recommendations suggest that penicillin, ampicillin, amoxicillin, tetracycline, and nonpotentiated sulfonamides also are poor choices for canine staphylococcal infection in Europe.[4-6,8]

Previous use of antibiotics negatively alters some sensitivity patterns. Staphylococcal sensitivity to ampicillin, amoxicillin, tetracycline, and nonpotentiated sulfonamides diminishes even further when previous antibiotic therapy has been utilized.[27,28,30] Sensitivity to erythromycin and lincomycin also diminishes when antibiotics have previously been given.[27,28,30] A recent study performed in the northeastern United States yielded the unexpected and surprising finding that *S. intermedius* isolated from dogs receiving multiple antibiotics prior to culture still maintained widespread sensitivity to erythromycin and tylosin, another macrolide![17] This finding is unexplained but suggests that differences in bacterial strains or markedly different antibiotic usage may lead to striking differences in susceptibility patterns in different regions of the world. Not unexpectedly, a recent study from England confirmed that multiresistant *S. intermedius* and gram-negative isolates were seen more commonly in referral practices than in general practice and that resistant bacterial populations were identified most frequently in specimens from deep pyoderma.[30]

Previous use of antibiotics apparently has less effect on sensitivity patterns of other antibiotics. Multiple studies indicate that trimethoprim- and ormetoprim-potentiated sulfonamides, oxacillin, clavulanic acid–potentiated amoxicillin, and cephalothin sensitivity patterns were

> In a recent study from England, resistant bacterial populations were identified most frequently in specimens from deep pyoderma.

not significantly altered by previous use.[11,16,28,30,33,34,36]

Multiple predictions have been made that antibiotic-resistant *S. intermedius* would preclude the use of many antibiotics commonly employed in the treatment of skin diseases. An examination of similarities and differences in antibiotic susceptibility patterns in studies published over the past two decades indicates that, remarkably, little change has occurred.[22,24-31] Somewhat surprisingly, strains of *S. intermedius* frequently encountered as pathogens in canine pyoderma apparently are no more resistant to commonly used antibiotics than they were 20 years ago.

Clinical Trials

Clinical trials have demonstrated that a wide range of different antibiotics are effective in managing various types of canine pyoderma.[32-38] Erythromycin, tylosin, lincomycin, clindamycin, chloramphenicol, trimethoprim- and ormetoprim-potentiated sulfonamides, oxacillin, cephalexin, cefadroxil, enrofloxacin, clavulanic acid–potentiated amoxicillin, and rifampin all have been either shown to be efficacious or have been more subjectively advocated.[1-12,14-17,21-38]

Kunkle and others recently published an epidemiologic study surveying adverse side effects seen with oral antibiotic therapy.[39] A significantly increased frequency of side effects was seen only with erythromycin in comparison with other orally administered antibiotics. Fifty-two percent of owners reported either vomiting, diarrhea, loss of appetite, depression, polyuria/polydipsia, or personality change as putative side effects of erythromycin administration.[39] Even considering a profound placebo effect, the percentage of perceived side effects was surprisingly high. Amoxicillin, lincomycin, and trimethoprim-sulfadiazine all caused significantly fewer side effects than did erythromycin. Trimethoprim-sulfadiazine, the most commonly used antibiotic in this study, did not cause a substantial number of adverse drug reactions.[39]

Rational Antibiotic Selection

Veterinary dermatologists select antibiotics for the management of canine pyoderma based on data from culture and sensitivity studies, clinical trials, review articles or book chapters, presentations at veterinary meetings, and past clinical experience as well as from objective and subjective preferences. All of the antibiotics mentioned as being efficacious (i.e., erythromycin, tylosin, lincomycin, clindamycin, chloramphenicol, trimethoprim- and ormetoprim-potentiated sulfonamides, oxacillin, cephalexin, cefadroxil, enrofloxacin, clavulanic acid–potentiated amoxicillin, and rifampin) have their devotees and detractors. The opinions expressed by the author in this section are personal preferences based on the assimilation of data (both valid and suspect) accrued in the practice of dermatology in California and Pennsylvania and are balanced by opinions of other veterinary dermatologists.

> Antibiotic therapy must be maintained until complete elimination of bacterial infection rather than simply transient remission is achieved.

There is almost universal agreement on which antibiotics *not* to use in the management of canine pyoderma. Penicillin, ampicillin, tetracycline, nonpotentiated sulfonamides, and amoxicillin should be avoided due to poor efficacy.[1-12,14]

Kwochka recently has recommended a complex tiered system for antibiotic usage based on previous response to antibiotics and severity and depth of infection. Erythromycin, lincomycin, and clindamycin are recommended for first-occurrence pyoderma, and trimethoprim-sulfadiazine, ormetoprim-sulfadimethoxine, and chloramphenicol are recommended for refractory pyoderma. β-Lactamase–resistant penicillins (oxacillin), amoxicillin-clavulanate, cephalosporins (cephalexin and cefadroxil), and rifampin are recommended for resistant infections and long-term maintenance of chronic recurrent pyoderma. Fluoroquinolones (enrofloxacin) and aminoglycosides are recommended for mixed infections.[7]

Scott, Miller, and Griffin have modified the tiered system of Kwochka. Their recommendations include chloramphenicol, clindamycin, erythromycin, lincomycin, and tylosin for first-occurrence pyoderma and ormetoprim-sulfadiazine, trimethoprim-sulfonamides (sulfadiazine or sulfamethoxazole), plus enrofloxacin for recurrent cases with previous antibiotic treatment. Amoxicillin-clavulanate, cefadroxil, cephalexin, cloxacillin, and oxacillin are listed for long-term use. Clindamycin, enrofloxacin, and rifampin (in conjunction with cephalexin or oxacillin) are listed for scarred pyoderma and interdigital granuloma, and enrofloxacin is listed for gram-negative rod pyoderma and otitis.[11]

DeBoer has suggested that trimethoprim-sulfadiazine, erythromycin, lincomycin, chloramphenicol, clindamycin, and ormetoprim-sulfadimethoxine should be used as first-line antibiotics. He lists oxacillin, cephalexin, and amoxicillin-clavulanate as excellent antibiotics, and fluoroquinolones (enrofloxacin and ciprofloxacin) and aminoglycosides as "effective but usually unnecessary antibiotics."[10] Mason and Moriello use cephalexin, clavulanic acid–potentiated amoxicillin, clindamycin, enrofloxacin, erythromycin, lincomycin, oxacillin, and trimethoprim-potentiated sulfonamides,[8,9] and Lloyd indicates similar preferences.[6]

Personal Preferences

The author has successfully used all of the antibiotics previously mentioned (with the exception of tylosin) for the management of canine pyoderma. Personal preferences are based on perceived efficacy, spectrum of activity, drug distribution, safety, lack of side effects, cost, route of administration, and required dosing frequency. Based on these criteria, the author's preferred narrow-spectrum antibiotics include **erythromycin, lincomycin,** and **oxacillin**. Preferred broader-spectrum antibiotics with excellent efficacy in canine pyoderma include **cephalexin, cefadroxil, ormetoprim-potentiated sulfonamides,** and **enrofloxacin** (Table 10-3). Other antibiotics are occasionally used or are recommended after consultations with clinicians on specific cases.

Owner compliance with different dosage regimens is not well studied in veterinary medicine. Differences in efficacy seen with various products may be partially due to differences in compliance. The author views drugs that need to be given only once or twice daily as having distinct advantages over drugs requiring owner administration three times daily. Indeed, owner schedules may preclude effective dosing three times a day, even with a conscientious owner. Only two antibiotics beneficial in the management of canine pyoderma may be administered once daily, **enrofloxacin** and **ormetoprim-potentiated sulfadimethoxine**. These drugs afford added convenience as well as potential increases in compliance. **Cephalexin, cefadroxil,** and **lincomycin** require dosing only twice daily. All other recommended antibiotics require administration three times daily.

The author recommends **erythromycin, lincomycin,** and **ormetoprim-potentiated sulfadimethoxine** for the management of uncomplicated, first-occurrence superficial pyoderma. Based on recent data, **tylosin** may be an interesting alternative,[17] especially because it can be administered only twice daily.

Erythromycin is a bacteriostatic macrolide available worldwide as a generic. The major advantages of erythromycin are cost (it is one of the least expensive antibiotics) and the rarity with which it produces side effects. Disadvantages include required dosing three times daily; a high frequency of vomiting, diarrhea, and other relatively minor side effects; and the potential for plasmid-mediated resistance developing rapidly after previous antibiotic use. Staphylococcal sensitivity to erythromycin seems to vary widely in different regions of the world. Cross-resistance is shared with other macrolides and lincomycin, precluding the use of other related drugs when the initial antibiotic is unsuccessful. Cost has led to the common usage of erythromycin, especially in larger dogs.

Lincomycin is macrolide-like lincosamide with a similar mode of action and identical patterns of sensitivity and resistance as erythromycin. Advantages of lincomycin are the twice-daily regimen and the rarity of gastrointestinal side effects, in contrast with erythromycin. Cost is the major disadvantage.

Ormetoprim-potentiated sulfadimethoxine is a comparatively new potentiated sulfonamide. Advantages include a once-daily dosing regimen and the likelihood that the drug has less potential for inducing either keratoconjunctivitis sicca or other more serious drug reactions than sulfadiazine-containing trimethoprim-potentiated sulfonamides. A

TABLE 10-3

ANTIBIOTICS USEFUL IN THE MANAGEMENT OF CANINE PYODERMA

- **NARROW-SPECTRUM**
  Erythromycin
  Lincomycin
  Oxacillin

- **BROAD-SPECTRUM**
  Cephalexin, cefadroxil
  Ormetoprim-potentiated sulfonamides
  Enrofloxacin

study evaluating tear production in 42 dogs receiving ormetoprim-potentiated sulfadimethoxine for 3 weeks found no significant differences in tear production.[39a]

Other possible candidates for the management of uncomplicated, first-occurrence pyoderma include **clindamycin** and **trimethoprim-potentiated sulfonamides**. Clindamycin is closely related to lincomycin and functions similarly, except for better absorption and tissue penetration. Unfortunately, clindamycin commonly is cost prohibitive.

Trimethoprim-potentiated sulfonamides exhibit good efficacy in the management of canine pyoderma. Advantages include twice-daily administration and cost, if generic trimethoprim-potentiated sulfamethoxazole is used. Veterinary brand name trimethoprim-sulfadiazine is a more expensive alternative. The efficacy of the various trimethoprim-potentiated sulfonamides seems comparable. The disadvantages of these products are of concern. Trimethoprim-potentiated sulfonamides are the most commonly recognized cause of cutaneous adverse drug reactions seen by the Dermatology Service at the University of California, Veterinary Medical Teaching Hospital.[40] Reactions range from minor papular rashes and erythema multiforme minor to life-threatening erythema multiforme major and toxic epidermal necrolysis. Nondermatologic adverse reactions include the induction of keratoconjunctivitis sicca by sulfadiazine-containing products. Trimethoprim-potentiated sulfadiazine is not recommended for use in Doberman pinschers because some members of this breed have a genetically enhanced susceptibility to adverse reactions. Susceptible Doberman pinschers may develop immune complex disease and nonseptic arthritis.[41,42] Similar reactions have been seen occasionally in a variety of other breeds. Although epidemiologic data from Kunkle and others[39] indicate that the actual frequency of adverse drug reactions to trimethoprim-potentiated sulfonamides is small, the striking and severe nature of the cutaneous adverse drug reactions seen with trimethoprim-sulfonamides has caused the author to reconsider recommending the use of this group of antibiotics.[40–42]

The author recommends the use of first-generation cephalosporins (**cephalexin** and **cefadroxil**), **enrofloxacin,** and **oxacillin** for pyoderma refractory to initial antibiotic therapy or recurrent pyoderma. Other veterinary dermatologists have had excellent success with **amoxicillin-clavulanate.** However, in the opinion of the author, considering both efficacy and cost, amoxicillin-clavulanate offers few advantages. Amoxicillin-clavulanate does become a more reasonable choice if long-term management with extended regimens is needed because suboptimal dosing does not result in resistance. Chronic, refractory, deep pyoderma frequently requires an antibiotic with superior penetrating ability because sequestered foci of infection and scarring may prevent access of the antibiotic to the actual sites of infection. Under these circumstances, **cephalexin** and **enrofloxacin** are the antibiotics of choice. On rare occasions, **rifampin** (in conjunction with cephalexin or oxacillin) may be used if the antibiotics mentioned above have not been successful.

Cephalexin is a broad-spectrum, first-generation bactericidal cephalosporin with excellent activity against *S. intermedius* and many secondary gram-negative invading organisms. Advantages include twice-daily administration, good tissue penetration, rarity of resistance, and moderate cost as a generic. The only disadvantage has been concern for the development of resistant bacteria. The prediction that widespread resistance develops with increased use has not materialized. **Cefadroxil** shares all the advantages of cephalexin except cost; consequently, it is used primarily in small dogs.

Enrofloxacin and other fluoroquinolones are new, broad-spectrum bactericidal antibiotics. Advantages include once-daily dosing, outstanding tissue penetration, activity against *S. intermedius* and multiple gram-negative secondary invading organisms, and rarity of resistance. Once-daily dosing is effective because the bacterial killing action is concentration rather than time dependent.[43] Potent tissue penetrating abilities are partially due to uptake of the drug by macrophages, leading to elevated concentrations in regions of chronic inflammation.[44–48] An intriguing possible added advantage beyond simply

> Enrofloxacin and ormetoprim-potentiated sulfadimethoxine are the only two antibiotics in the management of canine pyoderma that can be administered once daily.

biologically strategic localization of antibiotic would be the killing of staphylococci within macrophages of immunologically compromised dogs with defects in phagocytic killing ability.[44] Bacterial resistance is rare because it must be induced by genetic mutations instead of plasmid transference. Fluoroquinolones cannot be used in growing dogs because articular damage may occur. Otherwise, cost is the only disadvantage.

Extensive scar tissue with granulomatous inflammation separating and protecting sequestered foci of infection is seen in dogs with chronic, refractory deep pyoderma. **Enrofloxacin** and **cephalexin** are drugs of choice in these circumstances because they exhibit a broad spectrum of bactericidal activity. Enrofloxacin offers excellent tissue penetration, and cephalexin offers good penetrating ability.

Oxacillin is a β-lactamase–resistant, narrow-spectrum synthetic penicillin. Advantages include excellent efficacy in pyoderma without substantial scar tissue and a low frequency of side effects. The primary disadvantage, even as a generic, is cost. Oxacillin also must be administered three times daily. Because food interferes with absorption, oxacillin should be administered at least 1 hour before feeding.

Amoxicillin-clavulanate is somewhat popular as a broad-spectrum bactericidal antibiotic. Controversy still exists with respect to the appropriate dosage for canine pyoderma. Carlotti and Ovaert have reported that the manufacturer's dosage regimen is sufficient.[33] Other dermatologists, however, have suggested either much higher dosages or giving the drug three times daily, based on clinical failures.[7,8,10] A recent, blinded, multicenter comparison of two dose rates of amoxicillin-clavulanate in 68 dogs indicated that the manufacturer's recommended dosage was sufficient in most cases.[38]

Rifampin is a bactericidal antibiotic with potent initial activity against *S. intermedius* coupled with excellent ability to penetrate scar tissue. Unfortunately, resistance develops very rapidly, necessitating concurrent administration of β-lactamase–resistant antibiotics such as **cephalexin** or **oxacillin**. An additional major limiting factor besides rapid resistance is the potential for severe hepatotoxicity. Rifampin is contraindicated in patients with preexisting liver disease. Dogs receiving rifampin should have liver enzymes monitored at least every 2 weeks. Due to problems with toxicity and resistance, rifampin should be considered only after referral to a dermatologist and should not be considered as part of the normal armamentarium for the treatment of canine pyoderma.

Occasionally, extended regimens of antibiotics are warranted in the long-term management of recurrent canine pyoderma (see Chapter 13). This use of systemic antibiotics should be considered as a last resort. Antibiotics that have proven most effective for extended regimens include **cephalexin, enrofloxacin, oxacillin,** and **clavulanic acid–potentiated amoxicillin.** Extended regimens should only be implemented after the pyoderma has been brought under complete control by a standard course of appropriate antibiotics.

TOPICAL ANTIBACTERIAL THERAPY

Topical antibacterial therapy is useful in the management of all types of canine pyoderma. The rationale behind using antibacterial agents is that appropriate products will dramatically decrease the surface bacterial counts on skin and may limit the number of recolonizing organisms, thereby diminishing the likelihood of recurrence of infection. Topical therapy may be employed as a sole modality or may be used adjunctively, usually in conjunction with systemic antibiotics. An ideal topical product should aid in the initial resolution of the infection as well as aid in the prevention of relapses by limiting the bacterial surface flora for as long as possible.

Antibacterial agents can be classified as shampoos, whirlpools, soaks, rinses, sprays, lotions, gels, creams, and ointments. Shampoo is the most efficient and most commonly used topical delivery system for widespread canine pyoderma. Whirlpools or soaks are beneficial in removing debris and encouraging drainage in deep pyoderma. Antibacterial agents also may be useful in cream, ointment, or gel bases as sole therapy for more localized infection or adjunctively over limited areas.[14,49] Rinses are underutilized as a vehicle for antibacterial agents in veterinary dermatology.

Antibacterial Shampoo

Antibacterial shampoos offer the additional benefits of simple cleansing of the hair coat and underlying skin as well

> Shampoo is the most efficient and most commonly used topical delivery system for widespread canine pyoderma.

as removal of inflammatory products and other debris that can prevent drainage and encourage additional inflammation. Pain and pruritus may be reduced substantially. Improvement in patient attitude and owner encouragement because of the rapidity of response are less tangible additional benefits. The entire dog should be cleansed with the shampoo for a minimum of 10 minutes contact time.

Shampoo therapy may be used as an alternative to systemic antibiotics in some cases of surface pyoderma and is a beneficial adjunct in the management of superficial and deep pyoderma (see Chapters 6–8). All surface pyodermas (i.e., pyotraumatic dermatitis, intertrigo, and mucocutaneous pyoderma) benefit from antibacterial shampoos. Antibacterial shampoo may be used with antiinflammatory therapy (pyotraumatic dermatitis); before the application of topical antibacterial gels, creams, or ointments (intertrigo and mucocutaneous pyoderma); or in conjunction with systemic antibiotics (mucocutaneous pyoderma [see Chapter 6]). Antibacterial shampoos used as an adjunct to systemic antibiotic therapy speed resolution of both superficial and deep pyoderma (see Chapters 7 and 8). Antibacterial shampoo also may diminish the likelihood or frequency of recurrence of recurrent pyoderma (see Chapter 13).[50,51]

Antibacterial shampoos should be used a minimum of once weekly because none of the available products has a residual action for a duration of 1 week.[52] Twice-weekly shampoos are advantageous but time consuming for the owner. In dogs with deep pyoderma, antibacterial shampoos are used in conjunction with clipping and whirlpools or soaks. Dogs with deep pyoderma benefit from frequent (daily) antibacterial shampoo after clipping has removed matted hair and adherent debris.

Currently available antibacterial shampoos contain either benzoyl peroxide, benzoyl peroxide and sulfur, chlorhexidine, ethyl lactate, or triclosan. Benzoyl peroxide is the most commonly used agent in antibacterial shampoos. Beneficial features include potent antimicrobial action, follicular flushing, and keratolytic degreasing and comedolytic activity. Benzoyl peroxide may be especially useful in dogs with folliculitis and furunculosis because follicular flushing encourages drainage and removes sequestered purulent debris. Potential negative features of benzoyl peroxide use include irritation as well as drying and bleaching action on fabrics. Benzoyl peroxide is difficult to formulate and package without degradation to nonactive breakdown products. Consequently, generic products should be avoided, and the practice of buying in bulk and repackaging is not recommended. A controlled, quantitative study by Kwochka and Kowalski comparing the prophylactic activity of benzoyl peroxide, chlorhexidine, complexed iodine, and triclosan against *S. intermedius* demonstrated that benzoyl peroxide is clearly superior in preventing recolonization.[52] A variety of excellent products containing benzoyl peroxide are available internationally.[a–d] Benzoyl peroxide and sulfur offers an excellent combination with additional degreasing effects.[d]

Chlorhexidine is another antimicrobial agent formulated in shampoos. It is less irritating than benzoyl peroxide and offers an alternative for dogs that are especially sensitive to the irritation and dryness sometimes produced by benzoyl peroxide–containing products. Negative features are that chlorhexidine is a less potent antimicrobial agent than benzoyl peroxide and does not offer follicular flushing. Multiple products are available.[e,f]

Triclosan is less irritating than benzoyl peroxide but also has less antibacterial activity than either benzoyl peroxide or chlorhexidine and does not exhibit follicular flushing. Triclosan can be combined with sulfur and salicylic acid to add antibacterial activity to antiseborrheic shampoos.[g,h]

Ethyl lactate is a relatively new antibacterial agent with substantial promise.[53] Positive features include considerably less irritation than benzoyl peroxide coupled with good antibacterial potency. However, follicular flushing activity is not seen. Ethyl lactate shampoos offer a reasonable alternative in dogs sensitive to benzoyl peroxide.[i]

Antibacterial Soaks and Whirlpools

Dogs with deep pyoderma benefit from the cleansing and gentle debridement provided by whirlpools or soaks. After close clipping and shampooing, dogs with generalized deep pyoderma should be either soaked or whirlpooled in warm water containing antibacterials such as povidone-iodine or chlorhexi-

> Dogs with deep pyoderma benefit from the cleansing and gentle debridement provided by whirlpools or soaks.

dine. Foot soaks with the same active ingredients can be used for dogs with pedal folliculitis and furunculosis. If feasible, whirlpools should be used because the agitation they provide is superior to the effect of simple soaking. Soaks and whirlpools are labor intensive. Hospitalized dogs benefit from daily or twice-daily treatment for 15 to 30 minutes. Soaking can be accomplished by owners at home.

Antibacterial Gels, Creams, and Ointments

Gels, creams, and ointments containing antibacterial agents may be used to treat limited areas of infection. Cost, messiness, and time of application limit their usefulness when larger areas are involved. Pyoderma most amenable to treatment with agents in these vehicles include intertrigo, mucocutaneous pyoderma, muzzle folliculitis and furunculosis (canine acne), callus pyoderma, pyotraumatic folliculitis, and pedal folliculitis and furunculosis (see Chapters 6–8).

Benzoyl peroxide, also available in a gel formulation, is most useful in the management of intertrigo and muzzle folliculitis and furunculosis. Caution must be exercised in using benzoyl peroxide in a formulation designed to remain on the dog because permanent bleaching of fabric or carpeting can occur if dogs rub the residue on these materials. Multiple products are available.[j,k]

Mupirocin is a newer, novel antibacterial agent formed as a fermentation product of *Pseudomonas fluorescens*.[54] This potent topical antibiotic, available in a polyethylene glycol ointment base[l], is the first new topical antibiotic to be approved in the United States since neomycin in the 1950s. Many other countries have subsequently used fusidic acid as an additional potent topical antibacterial agent. Mupirocin inhibits bacterial protein synthesis and shows no cross-reactivity with any other group of antibiotics. Superior penetrating ability allows mupirocin to be used topically for deep as well as superficial pyoderma. The agent can be used in cases of intertrigo, mucocutaneous pyoderma, canine muzzle folliculitis and furunculosis, pedal folliculitis and furunculosis, callus pyoderma, and other pyodermas where a localized, penetrating topical antibacterial effect is desired. Mupirocin is not formulated for use on mucosal surfaces and is contraindicated in circumstances where absorption of large amounts of the polyethylene glycol vehicle is possible because of the potential of nephrotoxicity.[54]

IMMUNOMODULATORY THERAPY

Immunomodulatory therapy remains controversial in the management of canine pyoderma. However, various immunomodulatory preparations do enjoy popular support among veterinary dermatologists.[7,10,55] Controversy probably reflects perceived lack of efficacy, especially in general practice, and appropriate case selection. Even in successful cases, response to immunomodulatory therapy is seldom complete. Instead, the frequency or severity of infection is diminished. In the author's opinion, immunomodulation should be viewed predominantly as a therapeutic option for preventing recurrence of pyoderma rather than as a treatment for ongoing pyoderma. The author also believes that dogs with superficial pyoderma, such as superficial folliculitis and superficial spreading pyoderma, are more likely to benefit from immunomodulatory therapy than dogs with deep pyoderma.

Reports of poor efficacy from general practice may reflect case selection. If immunomodulatory therapy is used routinely as adjunctive therapy in the management of all pyodermas, results will be poor, leading to general dissatisfaction with this modality. Immunomodulatory therapy is most often successful in dogs with idiopathic recurrent superficial pyoderma (where underlying, predisposing diseases have not been identified) that respond completely to appropriate therapy, but recrudescence occurs within several weeks after discontinuing therapy. To date, no one has reported a method of predicting which types of idiopathic recurrent pyoderma are most likely to respond to immunomodulatory therapy.

Most discussions of efficacy have been either highly subjective or anecdotal because clinicians commonly use immunomodulatory therapy in conjunction with systemic antibiotics and topical antibacterial therapy. Appropriately controlled blinded trials are necessary to conclusively determine efficacy. However, controlled trials are difficult to perform because immunomodulatory therapy rarely is used alone.

> Dogs with superficial pyoderma are more likely to benefit from immunomodulatory therapy than dogs with deep pyoderma.

Bacterin Preparations

Preparations containing killed bacteria are the most commonly used immunomodulatory therapy in the management of canine pyoderma. Available commercial products contain either killed *Staphylococcus* or *Propionibacterium* (*Corynebacterium*) as the antigen. According to DeBoer, "30 to 50% of dogs with recurrent pyoderma ultimately benefit from bacterin treatment."[10]

The most commonly used commercial bacterin in the United States contains bacterial antigens from serotypes I and III of *Staphylococcus aureus* isolated from humans.[m] Staphylococci are lysed by a polyvalent *Staphylococcus* bacteriophage, and the final product is purified by ultrafiltration. This product contains large quantities of protein A, which probably is responsible for the immunostimulating effects. Double-blinded, placebo-controlled data reported by DeBoer and others indicate efficacy beyond placebo effect in approximately 40% of cases.[56] DeBoer injected the product subcutaneously using a dosage of 0.5 ml twice weekly. A commonly used alternative regimen utilizes injections of 1 ml given weekly. It is recommended to give the product for at least 10 weeks. Most clinicians continue therapy for 20 or 30 weeks to determine efficacy, since the product is packaged in 10-ml vials. Successful usage, as determined by a decrease in frequency or severity of pyoderma, usually indicates the need for lifelong therapy. DeBoer indicates that this product may be beneficial in up to 70% of cases of idiopathic recurrent superficial pyoderma.[10] Kwochka maintains that 30% to 40% of carefully screened cases will show some response and agrees that bacterins are more likely to be beneficial in superficial pyoderma.[7] The author believes that this product is the most effective and most convenient immunomodulatory preparation of bacterial origin currently available. Furthermore, it is the only product where efficacy has been documented by double-blinded, placebo-controlled studies.

Various other staphylococcal bacterins originally designed to be used in the management of bovine mastitis have been used to treat canine pyoderma. Available products either contain killed preparations of *S. aureus* alone or in conjunction with α and β toxoids of *Staphylococcus*.[n,o] Side effects such as localized swelling and pain at the injection site, fever, and general malaise are noted commonly with these products, limiting wide acceptance and usage. Critical evaluations of these products have not been performed.

Autogenous bacterins also have been advocated for the management of canine pyoderma. These preparations are made from the specific staphylococcal organisms isolated from a dog with pyoderma for use in that dog. Inactivation methodology is crucial in determining the potential success of an autogenous product because the process must kill the organism without disrupting antigenic determinants necessary to elicit the desired immune response. Anecdotal reports suggest that benefit has been seen with autogenous products, especially in the management of recurrent pedal folliculitis and furunculosis. However, controlled or blinded studies have not been performed

A bacterin prepared from cultures of *Propionibacterium acnes* is available as an immunostimulant for intravenous use only.[p] One paper indicates efficacy,[57] but conflicting results have been obtained by various veterinary dermatologists. The product is administered once or twice weekly IV, at doses between 0.25 ml to 2 ml, depending on body weight. The requirement of frequent intravenous administration has deterred common usage.

Nonbacterial Immunostimulants

Nonbacterial immunomodulatory therapy for pyoderma also is controversial in veterinary dermatology. Controlled, blinded studies have not been performed to determine efficacy. Most reports are anecdotal, similar to those for bacterially derived immunostimulants, because most clinicians use immunomodulatory drugs in conjunction with antibiotics and topical antibacterial therapy.

Levamisole, a levoisomer of tetramisole, is marketed as a vermifuge for use in large animals.[q,r] In addition to an antihelminthic effect, levamisole may alter lymphocyte and phagocyte immune function by modifying leukocyte intracellular cyclic nucleotides. Levamisole is believed to have a "window" effect, whereby dosages too high or too low will cause immunosuppression rather than immunostimulation. Sheep boluses are the most convenient, available form of the drug. The recommended dosage of

> Preparations containing killed bacteria are the most commonly used immunomodulatory therapy in the management of canine pyoderma.

levamisole is 2.2 mg/kg PO given every other day. Many dermatologists believe that some efficacy has occurred in isolated cases, but controlled studies have not been performed. The author believes that efficacy probably is less than 20%.

Cimetidine is an H_2 histamine receptor blocker developed for use in treating gastric ulcers in humans. Because lymphocytes have surface H_2 receptors, cimetidine theoretically could reduce immunosuppression by down-regulating suppressor T lymphocytes, thereby modulating cytokine production. Dosages of 3 to 4 mg/kg PO given twice daily for at least 10 weeks have been suggested.[7,10] Cimetidine seems to be relatively safe for use in the dog but is expensive. Controlled studies of efficacy have not been performed.

APPROPRIATE INITIAL MANAGEMENT

Systemic antibiotic therapy is required for the successful management of most cases of superficial and deep canine pyoderma. In deep pyoderma, or if immunodeficiency is suspected or confirmed as an underlying cause of disease, the selection of a bactericidal rather than a bacteriostatic antibiotic is indicated. Topical antibacterial shampoo therapy should be used as a beneficial adjunct. Antibacterial whirlpools or soaks also are useful in the management of deep pyoderma. Initial, preliminary investigation of obvious predisposing factors also is warranted (see Chapters 6–8).

A more detailed investigation of potential underlying causes should be made if appropriate, initial therapy is not successful or if the pyoderma recurs. Additional underlying causes and other factors complicating management must be investigated, and additional modalities of therapy should then be considered (see Chapters 11–13).

ASSESSMENT OF THERAPY

All dogs receiving systemic antibiotics for pyoderma should be reevaluated within 7 to 14 days. If substantial improvement is not noted, therapy and various factors complicating management should be reevaluated. The clinician initially should determine whether owner compliance has led to appropriate dosage during therapy. If compliance has been appropriate, evaluation of drug loss leading to inadequate dosage through vomition, inactivation by food, or malabsorption should be pursued. If owner compliance or patient factors have not led to drug failure, the clinician should reevaluate the choice of antibiotic. If the causes of treatment failure are not found, the clinician should address factors that can complicate successful management (see Chapter 11) or reevaluate the possibility of underlying disease (see Chapter 12). Clinicians should always maintain the flexibility to consider the possibility that their initial diagnosis of pyoderma was incorrect. Because other skin diseases may mimic each category of pyoderma, the differential diagnosis should be reevaluated (see Chapters 6–8). The possibility of referral to a veterinary dermatologist should be considered as an option each time clinical failure occurs.

---

[a]OxyDex, DVM Pharmaceuticals.
[b]Pyoben®, Allerderm/Virbac.
[c]Micro Pearls™ Benzoyl Peroxide Shampoo, Evsco Pharmaceuticals.
[d]Sulf/OxyDex, DVM Pharmaceuticals.
[e]Nolvasan®, Fort Dodge.
[f]ChlorhexiDerm, DVM Pharmaceuticals.
[g]SebaLyt, DVM Pharmaceuticals.
[h]SeboRx™, DVM Pharmaceuticals.
[i]Etiderm™, Allerderm/Virbac.
[j]Pyoben Gel®, Allerderm/Virbac.
[k]OxyDex Gel, DVM Pharmaceuticals.
[l]Bactoderm®, Pfizer Animal Health.
[m]Staphage Lysate (SPL)®, Delmont Laboratories.
[n]Staphoid® A-B, Coopers Animal Health.
[o]Lysigin®, Bio-Ceutic.
[p]ImmunoRegulin®, ImmunoVet.
[q]Tramisol®, Mallinckrodt Veterinary.
[r]Levasole®, Mallinckrodt Veterinary.

REFERENCES

1. Ihrke PJ, Halliwell REW, Deubler MJ: Canine pyoderma, in Kirk RW (ed): *Current Veterinary Therapy VI*. Philadelphia, WB Saunders, 1976, pp 513–519.
2. Ihrke PJ: The management of canine pyodermas, in Kirk RW (ed): *Current Veterinary Therapy VIII*. Philadelphia, WB Saunders, 1983, pp 505–517.
3. Kunkle GA: New considerations for rational antibiotic therapy of cutaneous staphylococcal infection in the dog. *Semin Vet Med Surg* 2:212–220, 1987.
4. Fourrier P, Carlotti D, Magnol J-P, et al: Les pyodermites du chien. *Prat Med Chirurg Anim Compag* 23(6): 1–539, 1988.
5. Mason IS: Canine pyoderma. *J Small Anim Pract* 32:381–386, 1991.
6. Lloyd DH: Therapy for canine pyoderma, in Kirk RW, Bonagura JD (eds): *Current Veterinary Therapy XI*. Philadelphia, WB Saunders, 1992, pp 539–544.
7. Kwochka KW: Recurrent pyoderma, in Griffin CE, Kwochka KW, MacDonald JM (eds): *Current Veterinary Dermatology*. St. Louis, Mosby–Year Book, 1993, pp 3–21.
8. Mason I: Antibacterial strategies, in Harvey RG, Mason IS (eds): *Manual of Small Animal Dermatology*. Gloucestershire, BSAVA Publications, 1993, pp 213–220.

9. Mason I, Moriello K: Management of infectious disorders, in Moriello K, Mason I (eds): *Handbook of Small Animal Dermatology*. Oxford, Pergamon, 1995, pp 287–294.
10. DeBoer DJ: Management of chronic and recurrent pyoderma in the dog, in Bonagura JD (ed): *Kirk's Current Veterinary Therapy XII*. Philadelphia, WB Saunders, 1995, pp 611–617.
11. Scott DW, Miller WH, Griffin CE: *Muller & Kirk's Small Animal Dermatology*, ed 5. Philadelphia, WB Saunders, 1995, pp 218–221, 280–328.
12. Ihrke PJ: Therapeutic strategies involving antimicrobial treatment of the skin in small animals. *JAVMA* 185:1165–1168, 1984.
13. Ayliffe TR: Penetration of tissue by antibiotics. *Vet Dermatol Newsletter* 5(2):33–37, 1980.
14. Ihrke PJ: Bacterial infections of the skin, in Greene CE (ed): *Infectious Diseases of the Dog and Cat*. Philadelphia, WB Saunders, 1990, pp 72–79.
15. Paradis M, Lemay S, Scott DW, Miller WH Jr: Efficacy of enrofloxacin in the treatment of canine bacterial pyoderma. *Vet Dermatol* 1:123–127, 1990.
16. Scott DW, Miller WH Jr, Wellington JR: The combination of ormetoprim and sulfadimethoxine in the treatment of pyoderma due to *Staphylococcus intermedius* infection in dogs. *Canine Pract* 18:29–33, 1993.
17. Scott DW, Miller WH, Cayatte SM, Bagladi MS: Efficacy of tylosin tablets for the treatment of pyoderma due to *Staphylococcus intermedius* infection in dogs. *Can Vet J* 35:617–621, 1994.
18. Greene CE, Ferguson DC: Antibacterial chemotherapy, in Greene CE (ed): *Infectious Diseases of the Dog and Cat*. Philadelphia, WB Saunders, 1990, pp 461–493.
19. Huber WG: Penicillins, tetracycline and aminoglycosides, macrolides, lincosamide, polymixins, chloramphenicol and other antibacterial agents, in Booth NH, McDonald LE (eds): *Veterinary Pharmacology and Therapeutics*, ed 6. Ames, IA, Iowa State University Press, 1988, pp 796–847.
20. Ford R, Aronson AL: Antimicrobial drugs and infectious diseases, in Davis LE (ed): *Handbook of Small Animal Therapeutics*. New York, Churchill Livingstone, 1985, pp 45–88.
21. Nesbitt GH, Schmitz JA: Chronic bacterial dermatitis and otitis: A review of 195 cases. *JAAHA* 13:442–450, 1977.
22. Rhoades HE: Sensitivity of bacteria to 16 antibiotic agents. *Vet Med Small Anim Clin* 74:976–979, 1979.
23. Marshall AB: Antibiotic therapy of small animal dermatitis. *Vet Dermatol Newsletter* 5(2):45–58, 1980.
24. Engvall A, Wierys M: Antibiogram and production of β-lactamase by canine isolates of *Staphylococcus aureus*. *Nord Vet Med* 34:441–448, 1982.
25. Phillips WE Jr, Williams BJ: Antimicrobial susceptibility patterns of canine *Staphylococcus intermedius* from veterinary clinical specimens. *Am J Vet Res* 45:2376–2379, 1984.
26. Cox HC, Hoskins JD, Roy AF: Antimicrobial susceptibility of coagulase-positive staphylococci isolated from Louisiana dogs. *Am J Vet Res* 45:2039–2042, 1984.
27. Medleau L, Long RE, Brown LJ, Miller WH Jr: Frequency and antimicrobial susceptibility of staphylococcal species isolate from canine pyodermas. *Am J Vet Res* 47:229–231, 1986.
28. Kunkle GA: Sensitivity of staphylococcal isolates in canine pyoderma. Proceedings of the American Academy of Veterinary Dermatology/American College of Veterinary Dermatology. Phoenix, Arizona, 1987, pp 6–7.
29. Devriese L: Antibiotic sensitivity and resistance of *Staphylococcus intermedius* strains isolated from dogs in Belgium. *Vlaams Diergeneesk Tijdschr* 57:40–45, 1988.
30. Noble WC, Kent LE: Antibiotic resistance in *Staphylococcus intermedius* isolated from cases of pyoderma in the dog. *Vet Dermatol* 3:71–74, 1992.
31. Reedy LM: Comparative results of 100 antibiotic sensitivity tests on *Staphylococcus intermedius* (1982–1994), in Proceedings of the Annual Meeting of the American Academy/College of Veterinary Dermatology, 1995, p 91.
32. Cannon RW: Clinical evaluation of Tribrissen®—A new antibacterial agent for dogs and cats. *Vet Med Small Anim Clin* 71:1090–1091, 1976.
33. Carlotti D, Ovaert P: Utilisation de l'association amoxycilline-acide clavulonique dans le traitement de pyodermites du chien. *Prat Med Chirurg Anim Compag* 23:519–522, 1988.
34. Guaguere E, Marc JP: Utilisation de la cefalexine dans le traitement des pyodermites. *Prat Med Chirurg Anim Compag* 24:124–129, 1989.
35. Angarano DW, MacDonald JM: Efficacy of cefadroxil in the treatment of bacterial dermatitis in dogs. *JAVMA* 194:57–59, 1989.
36. Frank LA, Kunkle GA: Comparison of the efficacy of cefadroxil and generic and proprietary cephalexin in the treatment of pyodermas in dogs. *JAVMA* 203:530–533, 1993.
37. Prost C, Arfi L: Utilisation de la lincomycine dans le traitement des pyodermites du chien. *Prat Med Chirurg Anim Compag* 28:495–498, 1993.
37a. Messinger LM, Beale KM: A blinded comparison of the efficacy of daily and twice daily trimethoprim-sulfadiazine and daily sulfamethoxine-ormetoprim therapy in the treatment of canine pyoderma. *Vet Dermatol* 4(1):13–18, 1993.
38. Lloyd DH, Carlotti DN, Koch H, Halliwell REW: Clavulanate-potentiated amoxicillin in the treatment of canine pyodermas: Comparison of two dose rates. Proceedings of the European Society of Veterinary Dermatology, Bordeau, 1994, p 63.
39. Kunkle GA, Sundlof S, Deisling K: Adverse side effects of oral antibacterial therapy in dogs and cats: An epidemiologic study of pet owners' observations. *JAAHA* 31:46–55, 1995.
39a. Mueller RS, Bettenay S, Ihrke PJ: Unpublished data, 1992.
40. Ihrke PJ: Adverse drug reactions in dermatology. AAHA 61th Annual Meeting, Scientific Proceedings, 1994, pp 180–183.
41. Werner LL, Bright JM: Drug-induced immune hypersensitivity disorders in two dogs treated with trimethoprim sulfadiazine. *JAAHA* 19:783–790, 1983.
42. Giger U, Werner LL, Millichamp BVM, Gorman NT: Sulfadiazine-induced allergy in six Doberman pinschers. *JAVMA* 186:479–484, 1985.
43. Meinen JB, Rosen E, McClure JT: Pharmacodynamics of enrofloxacin in *Escherichia coli* and Staphylococcal infections. Proceedings of the American College of Veterinary Surgeons, 1995, p 67.
44. Easmon CSF, Crane JP: Uptake of ciprofloxacin by macrophages. *J Clin Pathol* 38:442–444, 1985.
45. Bryant RE, Mazza JA: Effect of abscess environment on the antimicrobial activity of ciprofloxacin. *Am J Med* 87(Suppl 5A):23s–27s, 1989.
46. Tulkens PM: Accumulation and subcellular distribution of antibiotics in macrophages in relation to activity against intracellular bacteria, in Fass RJ (ed): *Ciprofloxacin in Pulmonology*. Bern, W Zuckschwerdt Verlag Munchen, 1990, pp 12–20.
47. Nix DE, Goodwin SD, Peloquin CA, et al: Antibiotic tissue penetration and its relevance: Impact of tissue penetration on infection response. *Antimicrob Agents Chemother* 35:1953–1959, 1991.
48. Nikaido H, Thanassi DG: Penetration of lipophilic agents with multiple protonation sites into bacterial cells: Tetracyclines and fluoroquinolones as examples. *Antimicrob Agents Chemother* 37:1393–1399, 1993.
49. Ihrke PJ: Antibacterial therapy in dermatology, in Kirk RW (ed): *Current Veterinary Therapy IX*. Philadelphia, WB Saunders, 1986, pp 566–571.
50. Lloyd DH, Reyss-Brion A: Le peroxide de benzoyle: Efficacite clinique et bacteriologique dans le traitement des pyodermites chroniques. *Prat Med Chirurg Anim Compag* 19:445–448, 1984.
51. Ihrke PJ, Gross TL: Canine mucocutaneous pyoderma, in Bonagura JD (ed): *Kirk's Current Veterinary Therapy XII*. Philadelphia, WB Saunders, 1995, pp 618–619.
52. Kwochka KW, Kowalski JJ: Prophylactic efficacy of four antibacterial shampoos against *Staphylococcus intermedius* in dogs. *Am J Vet Res* 52:115–118, 1991.
53. Ascher F, Maynard L, Laurent J, Goubet B:: Controlled trials of ethyl lactate and benzoyl peroxide shampoos in the management of canine surface pyoderma and superficial pyoderma, in Von Tscharner C, Halliwell REW (eds): *Advances in Veterinary Dermatology*, vol 1. London, Baillière Tindall, 1990, pp 375–382.
54. Leyden JJ: Mupirocin: A new topical antibiotic. *J Am Acad Dermatol* 22:879–883, 1990.
55. Ihrke PJ: Antibiotic therapy and strategies for the management of recurrent pyoderma. Proceedings of the Nineteenth World Small Animal Veterinary Association Congress, Durban, South Africa, 1994, pp 241–245.
56. DeBoer DJ, Moriello KA, Thomes CB, et al: Evaluation of a commercial staphylococcal bacterin for management of idiopathic recurrent superficial pyoderma in dogs. *Am J Vet Res* 51:636-639, 1990.
57. Becker AM, Janik TA, Smith EK, et al: *Propionibacterium acnes* immunotherapy in chronic canine pyoderma. *J Vet Intern Med* 3:26–30, 1989.

Chapter 11

Factors Complicating Management of Pyoderma

The management of canine pyoderma can be complicated by various factors that can greatly influence prognosis. Inappropriate initial therapy, unidentified coexisting problems, sequestered foci of infection in deep pyoderma, and external environmental factors that may not be known to the veterinarian most commonly complicate management of pyoderma.[1-5] If these factors occur and are not identified and appropriately managed, either therapy will be unsuccessful or recurrence will ensue.

INAPPROPRIATE INITIAL THERAPY

Treatment failure and disease recurrence are most often associated with inappropriate initial therapy. Errors commonly are made in antibiotic selection, dosage used, and duration of therapy.[1-8] Antibiotics chosen empirically should have a known spectrum of activity against canine *Staphylococcus intermedius*, and data should be available indicating clinical efficacy in canine pyoderma (see Chapter 10). Many systemic antibiotics need to be dosed within a relatively narrow window, but underdosing is of greater importance because it can lead to diminished therapeutic efficacy. Overdosing is more likely to induce adverse reactions and may needlessly increase expense. Underdosing is common in large dogs, whereas overdosing is more common in very small dogs. Antibiotics should always be used for a minimum of 14 days in the management of canine pyoderma. In general, systemic antibiotics should be continued for a minimum of 1 week beyond clinical cure in superficial pyoderma and 2 weeks beyond clinical cure in deeper infections. Longer courses of antibiotic therapy contingent on the specific subgroup of pyoderma may be required (see Chapters 6–8). If initial therapy seemed appropriate after reevaluation, other potential factors complicating management should be reinvestigated.

COEXISTING PROBLEMS

The lack of identification of underlying diseases or circumstances that can contribute to pyoderma is an additional frequent cause of either initial treatment failure or recrudescence.[5,6,8,9] Problems commonly complicating management in this manner include underlying pruritic diseases (especially ectoparasitic hypersensitivities and other allergies), diseases altering the structure or function of the hair follicles, chronic cutaneous inflammation of any origin, and diseases that diminish immune surveillance against bacterial invasions such as endogenous or iatrogenic hyperglucocorticoidism and hypothyroidism (Table 11-1).

Underlying diseases that commonly induce recurrent skin infections in the dog are addressed in greater detail in Chapter 13.

SEQUESTERED FOCI OF INFECTION

Sequestered foci of bacterial infection are a common cause of either unsuccessful initial therapy or recurrence of canine deep pyoderma. Keratin debris from ruptured hair follicles encourages a foreign body granulomatous response in cases of deep pyoderma. This "walling off" of infected tissue can impede antibiotic penetration. Antibiotics of the penicillin family also are less effective when necrotic tissue and obstructed

> Treatment failure and disease recurrence are most often associated with inappropriate initial therapy.

TABLE 11-1
COEXISTING PROBLEMS COMMONLY COMPLICATING MANAGEMENT OF CANINE PYODERMA

- Underlying pruritic diseases (especially ectoparasitic hypersensitivities and other allergies)
- Diseases altering the structure or function of the hair follicles
- Chronic cutaneous inflammation of any origin
- Diseases that diminish immune surveillance against bacterial invasions such as endogenous or iatrogenic hyperglucocorticoidism and hypothyroidism

---

drainage routes create conditions that are no longer favorable for bacterial replication.[4,5,10]

Despite the greater accessibility of referable information to drug availability, sequestration, and elimination, most antibiotic dosages used in the treatment of canine pyoderma still are largely empiric. Because of the foreign body granulomatous response commonly initiated in cases of deep pyoderma and the resultant sequestered foci of infection, higher doses may be warranted in the management of chronic deep pyoderma.

EXTERNAL FACTORS

External environmental, social, and societal factors that influence therapeutic success rates have attracted greater scrutiny in human medicine in the past decade. Owner compliance, vomition of drug, and possible drug inactivation all may markedly affect therapeutic success rates.[1-10] Owner compliance is a problem largely unexplored in veterinary medicine. In human medicine, it is recognized that only 40% of prescriptions are even filled and only 40% or less of medication received is taken appropriately. Can we assume that circumstances are better in veterinary medicine? Most likely, compliance is better when owners are allotted drugs that need to be administered only once or even twice daily to their pets. This may contribute to a perceived enhanced efficacy in once-daily antibiotics such as ormetoprim-potentiated sulfadimethoxine and enrofloxacin. Twice-daily products such as cephalexin and lincomycin may offer advantages over antibiotics that require administration three times daily.

REFERENCES

1. Ihrke PJ: The management of canine pyodermas, in Kirk RW (ed): *Current Veterinary Therapy VIII*. Philadelphia, WB Saunders, 1983, pp 505–517.
2. Ihrke PJ: Antibacterial therapy in dermatology, in Kirk RW (ed): *Current Veterinary Therapy IX*. Philadelphia, WB Saunders, 1986, pp 566–571.
3. White SD, Ihrke PJ: Pyoderma, in Nesbitt GH (ed): *Dermatology—Contemporary Issues in Small Animal Practice*. New York, Churchill Livingstone, 1987, pp 95–121.
4. Ihrke PJ: An overview of bacterial skin disease in the dog. *Br Vet J* 433: 112–118, 1987.
5. Ihrke PJ: Bacterial infections of the skin, in Greene CE (ed): *Infectious Diseases of the Dog and Cat*. Philadelphia, WB Saunders, 1990, pp 72–79.
6. Scott DW, Miller WH, Griffin CE: *Muller & Kirk's Small Animal Dermatology*, ed 5. Philadelphia, WB Saunders, 1995, pp 55–173.
7. DeBoer DJ: Management of chronic and recurrent pyoderma in the dog, in Kirk RW (ed): *Current Veterinary Therapy IX*. Philadelphia, WB Saunders, 1995, pp 611–617.
8. Mason IS: Canine pyoderma. *J Small Anim Pract* 32:381–386, 1991.
9. Ihrke PJ: Current overview of the management of canine pyoderma. Proceedings of the Twentieth World Small Animal Veterinary Association Congress and the Twenty-fifth World Veterinary Association Congress, Yokohama, Japan. In press, 1995.
10. Ihrke PJ: Therapeutic strategies involving antimicrobial treatment of the skin in small animals. *JAVMA* 185:1165–1168, 1984.

Chapter 12

Canine Recurrent Pyoderma

GENERAL CONSIDERATIONS

Most patients with canine pyoderma respond appropriately and completely to initial therapeutic management. The original infection does not become chronic or recur after successful therapy has been completed. An unknown percentage of dogs with pyoderma recrudesce after apparent complete recovery.[1-5] These cases of recurrent pyoderma are among the most frustrating skin diseases in both general and specialty referral small animal practices.

Recurrent pyoderma may be defined as a bacterial skin infection that responds completely to appropriate systemic and topical antibacterial therapy, leaving the dog free of clinical signs of pyoderma and apparently normal or near normal between episodes of infection. Most cases of recurrent canine pyoderma occur secondary to underlying disease (Table 12-1), which can either be another skin disease or an underlying internal medical abnormality that increases the likelihood of the development of a secondary pyoderma. Recurrent pyoderma secondary to continuing, underlying skin disease may alter the clinical appearance of the underlying skin disease such that identification of the predisposing disease is more difficult until appropriate therapy for pyoderma has removed the visual signs of the secondary pyoderma. Consequently, the diagnosis of the underlying disease may be facilitated by an appropriate course of systemic antibiotics. Recurrent pyoderma is termed *idiopathic* only if *all* appropriate diagnostic tests have failed to reveal a predisposing cause, either dermatologic or nondermatologic, for the recurrent pyoderma in question.

The presence or absence of pruritus either directly attributable to the pyoderma or initiated by an underlying, predisposing disease is a critical feature in the effective diagnosis and management of canine recurrent pyoderma. If pruritus seen with a recurrent pyoderma is totally ameliorated by successful antibiotic therapy, it probably was caused by the bacterial infection. Conversely, if pruritus is still present after complete clinical resolution of the bacterial infection, it is most likely due to an underlying pruritic disease not yet diagnosed.

Similar to all types of pyoderma, recurrent pyoderma may be categorized as surface, superficial, or deep. Recurrence is the rule rather than the exception with canine surface pyoderma. In general, underlying causes are more readily identified with surface pyoderma, and initial therapy commonly includes management of predisposing causes. Consequently, recurrence of surface pyoderma is viewed as expected and therefore is not usually addressed in discussions of "recurrent pyoderma." Recurrent superficial pyoderma is the most common canine recurrent bacterial skin infection. Recurrent deep pyoderma is substantially less common. In the author's experience, many apparently recurrent deep pyodermas are, in actuality, cases in which complete cure has never been achieved and sequestered foci of infection remained after apparent clinical cure.

GENERAL CAUSES OF RECURRENT PYODERMA

Some generalizations can be made about the underlying causes of recurrent pyoderma. DeBoer has subdivided the underlying possible causes of recurrent (and chronic) canine pyoderma into

> Identification of persistent underlying skin disease is the single most useful process in diminishing the likelihood that pyoderma will recur.

TABLE 12-1
UNDERLYING DISEASES ASSOCIATED WITH RECURRENT CANINE PYODERMA

Nonparasitic allergic diseases	Atopic dermatitis Food allergy
Allergic parasitic diseases	Flea allergy dermatitis Cheyletiellosis Sarcoptic acariasis
Other parasitic diseases	Demodicosis
Endocrine diseases	Hypothyroidism Iatrogenic hyperglucocorticoidism Pituitary-dependent hyperadrenocorticism
Diseases of cornification	Primary keratinization defects Secondary "seborrhea"
Other infectious diseases	*Malassezia* dermatitis Dermatophytosis
Genodermatoses	Follicular dysplasia Color dilution alopecia
Other inflammatory diseases affecting hair follicles	Sebaceous adenitis
Occult neoplasia	Solar-induced squamous cell carcinoma

Immunodeficiency	Congenital
	Acquired
	  Systemic disease
	  Neoplasia
	  Immunosuppressive therapy

persistent underlying skin disease, bacterial hypersensitivity, immunodeficiency, resistant strains of *Staphylococcus intermedius*, and nonstaphylococcal pyoderma.[4] Among these possible underlying causes, persistent underlying skin disease is the most commonly documented underlying cause of recurrent pyoderma[2-5] (Table 12-2).

Persistent Underlying Skin Disease

Allergy (both parasitic and nonparasitic), diseases of cornification, endocrinopathies, other infections, physical trauma, and other less common skin diseases can predispose dogs to recurrent canine pyoderma. Identification of persistent underlying skin disease is the single most useful process in diminishing the likelihood that pyoderma will recur.

Underlying skin diseases predisposing dogs to recurrent pyoderma can be divided conveniently into pruritic and nonpruritic diseases. The presence or absence of pruritus after pyoderma has been eliminated is a key feature in the prioritization and differentiation of underlying causes of recurrent canine pyoderma. If an underlying pruritic disease is not diagnosed (pruritus of unknown origin), management of recurrent pyoderma may be very frustrating.

Concurrent pruritus strongly suggests the possibility of underlying allergic disease. Most pruritic ectoparasitic diseases (with the exception of demodicosis) probably are caused by allergy to the parasite or the waste products of the parasite. Atopic dermatitis, flea allergy dermatitis, and food allergy are common pruritic causes of recurrent pyoderma.

Canine atopic dermatitis is one of the most consistently documented underlying causes of recurrent pyoderma.[1-5] Increased staphylococcal adherence to corneocytes and enhanced absorption of protein A in atopic dogs could explain increased susceptibility to infection in dogs with this disease.[6-8]

Flea allergy dermatitis is the most common parasitic hypersensitivity that initiates recurrent pyoderma. Other ectoparasitic diseases such as cheyletiellosis occasionally may cause recurrent pyoderma. Although sarcoptic acariasis (canine scabies) may cause recurrent pyoderma, this combination probably is rare because obvious primary skin lesions allowing diagnosis remain after antibiotic therapy has removed the secondary pyoderma.

The injudicious use of glucocorticoids is an additional significant contributing factor in the induction of recurrent pyoderma in dogs with pruritic skin disease. Kwochka has stated that "the major predisposing factors [for recurrent pyoderma] in most parts of the United States are allergic dermatitis and long-term administration of glucocorticoids."[2] In fact, these two major predisposing factors commonly are combined in most cases where putative underlying causes can be identified.

Occult demodicosis is an additional parasitic cause of recurrent pyoderma. Recurrent deep pyoderma commonly occurs secondary to undiagnosed demodicosis, indicating the importance of skin scrapings in all cases of deep pyo-

TABLE 12-2
POSSIBLE CAUSES OF RECURRENT PYODERMA

- Persistent underlying skin disease
- Bacterial hypersensitivity
- Immunodeficiency
- Resistant strains of *Staphylococcus intermedius*
- Nonstaphylococcal pyoderma

derma. Demodicosis in long-coated breeds may not cause substantial alopecia, commonly lowering the index of suspicion for demodicosis.

Defects in cornification (seborrhea) can be both a pruritic and a nonpruritic cause of recurrent pyoderma. Qualitative and quantitative differences in surface bacterial flora are prominent features in dogs with cornification abnormalities.[9-11] Chronic inflammation with an abnormal surface flora probably contributes to recurrent bacterial infections. As in all underlying diseases that initiate recurrent pyoderma, treatment of the pyoderma facilitates identification of the underlying disease.

Endocrine diseases such as hypothyroidism, pituitary-dependent hyperadrenocorticism, and iatrogenic hyperglucocorticoidism may be responsible for initiating recurrent pyoderma even if there are minimal clinical signs referable to the underlying disease. Consequently, these diseases must be ruled out before dogs that appear clinically normal are diagnosed as having idiopathic recurrent pyoderma. Pruritus may be a feature of hypothyroidism if skin changes have become sufficiently chronic.

Genodermatoses causing anatomic abnormalities of the hair follicles may predispose dogs to recurrent superficial or deep infection. Examples of underlying genodermatoses that predispose dogs to recurrent pyoderma include follicular dysplasia and color dilution alopecia. Because clinically visible lesions may be subtle, the importance of skin biopsy as an imperative diagnostic tool is underscored.

Other inflammatory diseases affecting the hair follicle, such as sebaceous adenitis, also may predispose dogs to recurrent secondary pyoderma. A knowledge of frequently affected breeds (e.g., standard poodle, Akita, vizla, Samoyed) should increase index of suspicion; skin biopsy is confirmatory. Infectious inflammatory skin diseases such as *Malassezia* dermatitis and dermatophytosis rarely initiate recurrent pyoderma.

Dogs with occult neoplasia, such as solar-induced squamous cell carcinoma, may be presented as having recurrent pyoderma localized to thin-skinned, sparsely pigmented, or comparatively glabrous exposed regions of the body such as the ventral and lateral abdomen, lateral body wall, or face. Index of suspicion should be greater in regions of the world with substantial sun exposure, especially in predisposed breeds such as the dalmatian, bullterrier, greyhound, whippet, and Italian greyhound. Skin biopsy confirms the diagnosis.

Bacterial Hypersensitivity

Bacterial hypersensitivity as a perpetuator of chronic and recurrent canine pyoderma remains controversial in veterinary dermatology (see Chapter 3). Fadok and Edwards have speculated that hypersensitivity to bacterial super-antigens may play a role in the severe inflammation seen with some types of canine pyoderma.[12] Earlier preliminary data by Halliwell demonstrated higher levels of antistaphylococcal immunoglobulin E in dogs with recurrent pyoderma and erythematous spreading lesions.[13] A recent larger study by Morales, Schultz, and DeBoer substantiated an association between antistaphylococcal antibodies and various subgroups of canine pyoderma.[14] Although direct evidence showing a causal relationship has not been established, some of the severe, self-perpetuating inflammation and pruritus seen in dogs with pyoderma is likely due to a hypersensitivity reaction.

Immunodeficiency

Despite its attractiveness as a concept, generalized immunodeficiency is a rare cause of recurrent pyoderma. The few dogs seen by the author determined to have putative cellular immune dysfunction documented by lymphocyte blastogenesis have had predominantly chronic, deep pyoderma. Severe circulating immunoglobulin A (IgA) deficiency has been reported as a

> Despite its attractiveness as a concept, generalized immunodeficiency is a rare cause of recurrent pyoderma.

cause of both skin and respiratory infections. Currently, IgA deficiency is viewed as a rare and somewhat controversial cause of recurrent pyoderma.

Resistant Strains of *Staphylococcus intermedius*

Resistant strains of *Staphylococcus intermedius* are a very rare and commonly overdiagnosed cause of chronic and recurrent canine pyoderma. Although resistance frequently can occur to first-line antibiotics, canine strains of *S. intermedius* have shown a remarkable propensity *not* to develop resistance to antibiotics such as the cephalosporins, β-lactamase–resistant penicillins, and the fluoroquinolones.

Nonstaphylococcal Pyoderma

Canine pyoderma initiated by primary organisms other than *S. intermedius* is exceedingly rare (see Chapter 2). The culture of organisms other than *S. intermedius* commonly indicates the presence of secondary invaders or environmental contamination of the culture (see Chapter 9).

RECURRENT SURFACE PYODERMA

The term *surface pyoderma* encompasses pyotraumatic dermatitis (acute moist dermatitis, hot spots), intertrigo (skin-fold pyoderma, skin-fold dermatitis), and mucocutaneous pyoderma. Because surface pyoderma is largely a classification of convenience and most bacterial involvement probably is secondary, it is not surprising that the identified underlying causes of recurrent surface pyoderma are somewhat different from those seen in both superficial and deep pyoderma (Table 12-3).

The diagnosis of underlying predisposing abnormalities initiating pyotraumatic dermatitis and intertrigo is considered routine and rarely is problematic diagnostically because most pyotraumatic dermatitis is seen secondary to flea allergy dermatitis, and intertrigo correlates directly with the presence of an abnormal skin fold. Conversely, the underlying causes of recurrent mucocutaneous pyoderma are not known.

Pyotraumatic dermatitis develops secondary to underlying pruritic, allergic skin disease and resultant self-trauma. Focally directed self-trauma creates dramatic secondary lesions. Flea allergy dermatitis is the most common underlying,

TABLE 12-3
UNDERLYING CAUSES OF RECURRENT SURFACE PYODERMA

- **PYOTRAUMATIC DERMATITIS**
  Flea allergy dermatitis
  Atopic dermatitis
  Food allergy

- **INTERTRIGO**
  Breed-specific anatomic skin folds on lips, face, and tail
  Obesity-related

- **MUCOCUTANEOUS PYODERMA**
  Underlying causes not identified

initiating cause of most cases of canine pyotraumatic dermatitis. Much less commonly, other allergic diseases such as canine atopic dermatitis and food allergy have been implicated in initiating pyotraumatic dermatitis. Failure to adequately manage underlying allergic disease routinely results in recurrent pyotraumatic dermatitis. Pyotraumatic dermatitis secondary to flea allergy dermatitis has a marked site predilection for the dorsal lumbosacral region (see Chapter 6).

Intertrigo is seen in conjunction with specific anatomic abnormalities that are either breed standards or exaggerated expressions of breed standards. Bacterial involvement is secondarily associated with chronic friction, poor drainage leading to retention of secretions and excretions, and maceration at the sites of skin folding. Lip-fold, facial-fold, and tail-fold intertrigo have marked breed predilections. Lip-fold intertrigo is seen predominantly in springer spaniels, cocker spaniels, Saint Bernards, and Irish setters; facial-fold intertrigo is seen in brachycephalic breeds such as the Pekingese, pug, and English bulldog. Vulvar-fold intertrigo and obesity-fold intertrigo are both linked to obesity. Generalized fold intertrigo is seen in the Chinese shar-pei, predominantly in dogs with excessive wrinkling and prob-

> **Failure to adequately manage underlying allergic disease routinely results in recurrent pyotraumatic dermatitis.**

ably in association with abnormal production and accumulation of dermal mucin.

Mucocutaneous pyoderma is a poorly understood syndrome that predominantly involves the lips and perioral skin. Although recurrence is common, underlying causes have not been identified (see Chapter 6).

RECURRENT SUPERFICIAL PYODERMA

Most pyodermas classified as *recurrent* are superficial pyodermas. All three subgroupings of superficial pyoderma (impetigo, superficial folliculitis, and superficial spreading pyoderma) can become recurrent (Table 12-4).

Recurrence is infrequent in the most common form of bacterial impetigo seen in prepubescent and pubescent dogs; however, it is possible if putative triggering mechanisms such as fecal debris, urine scalding, hair coat matting, ectoparasitism, environmental hygiene, or poor nutrition are not managed concurrently. Recurrence is a frequent feature of the bullous form of impetigo seen in older dogs in conjunction with underlying immunosuppression. Recurrent bullous impetigo is evident most frequently with naturally occurring or iatrogenic hyperglucocorticoidism but also has been seen in association with diabetes mellitus, hypothyroidism, lymphoid neoplasia, and other less common debilitating or immunocompromising diseases.[15,16]

Recurrent superficial folliculitis is the most common recurrent pyoderma. The same underlying factors that cause superficial folliculitis to be the most common canine bacterial skin disease probably also contribute to recurrent superficial folliculitis being the most common recurrent canine bacterial skin disease. As discussed in Chapter 3, previously existing inflammation or hair follicle abnormalities including obstruction, atrophy, dysplasia, or degeneration predispose dogs to secondary bacterial folliculitis. In addition, these same ongoing abnormalities probably predispose dogs to recurrence unless the underlying problem is managed appropriately.

Canine atopic dermatitis is one of the most consistently important underlying causes of recurrent superficial folliculitis.[1-5] Superficial folliculitis also is seen secondary to other allergic or parasitic skin diseases. Defects of cornification (seborrhea) are other common initiators of recurrent superficial folliculitis. In addition, underlying pruritic skin disease from any etiology commonly predisposes dogs to recurrent superficial folliculitis. If the underlying pruritic disease is managed symptomatically with corticosteroids, the likelihood of recurrent pyoderma is increased.

Recurrent superficial spreading pyoderma also is common, either alone or in conjunction with superficial folliculitis. The same underlying causes that contribute to recurrent superficial folliculitis may be partly responsible for recurrent superficial spreading pyoderma.

RECURRENT DEEP PYODERMA

Although recurrent deep pyodermas are substantially less common than recurrent superficial pyodermas, the most commonly identified underlying causes are similar. As discussed previous-

TABLE 12-4
UNDERLYING CAUSES OF RECURRENT SUPERFICIAL PYODERMA

- **BULLOUS IMPETIGO**
  Hyperglucocorticoidism
  Diabetes mellitus
  Hypothyroidism
  Lymphoid neoplasia
  Other immunocompromising diseases

- **SUPERFICIAL FOLLICULITIS AND SUPERFICIAL SPREADING PYODERMA**
  Canine atopic dermatitis
  Other allergic diseases
  Parasitic diseases
  Seborrhea
  Other underlying pruritic skin diseases
  Abnormalities of hair follicles

> Labeling of a recurrent pyoderma as idiopathic implies that the prognosis for complete cure is poor, and the goal of therapy will most likely be to control rather than cure the infection.

ly in Chapter 8, the reasons why some superficial pyodermas proceed to involve deeper structures are largely unknown. Care must be taken to differentiate true recurrent deep pyoderma from chronic deep pyoderma in cases where complete resolution has not been achieved.

Occult demodicosis is a much more common underlying cause of deep pyoderma than of superficial pyoderma. Recurrent deep pyoderma after apparent clinical cure should increase suspicion for underlying demodicosis, especially if uncommon sites for primary pyoderma such as the face, lateral trunk, and dorsal trunk are affected. Deep pyoderma secondary to demodicosis obviously follows the breed predilections of the underlying demodicosis.

Kwochka notes that chronic, relapsing deep pyoderma is more common in short-coated breeds. He speculates that this may be caused by a more intense foreign body reaction to keratin.[2] Short-coated dogs at apparent increased risk for relapsing deep pyoderma include bullterrier breeds, dalmatians, Doberman pinschers, and Great Danes.[16]

Breed predilections can markedly increase suspicion for underlying diseases (see Chapter 8). For example, recurrent deep pyoderma in an Akita suggests underlying sebaceous adenitis; recurrent deep pyoderma located in the appropriate sites in a dalmatian, bullterrier, greyhound, whippet, or Italian greyhound should increase suspicion for underlying occult solar-induced neoplasia. Recurrent callus pyoderma in large, short-coated breeds should initiate attempts to diminish recurrent trauma to the affected pressure points.

IDIOPATHIC RECURRENT PYODERMA

The term *idiopathic* should be used to describe recurrent pyoderma only after all possible underlying causes that usually initiate recurrent bacterial infections are eliminated. The performance of all appropriate diagnostic tests should be emphasized to the owner because the identification of underlying causes substantially enhances the likelihood of complete clinical cure. The owner should be informed that the labeling of a recurrent pyoderma as idiopathic implies that the prognosis for complete cure is poor, and the goal of therapy will most likely be to control rather than cure the infection (see Chapter 13).

REFERENCES

1. DeBoer DJ: Strategies for management of recurrent pyoderma in dogs, in DeBoer DJ (ed): *Veterinary Clinics of North America: Advances in Clinical Dermatology.* Philadelphia, WB Saunders, 1990, pp 1509–1524.
2. Kwochka KW: Recurrent pyoderma, in Griffin CE, Kwochka KW, MacDonald JM (eds): *Current Veterinary Dermatology.* St. Louis, Mosby–Year Book, 1993, pp 3–21.
3. Ihrke PJ: Antibiotic therapy and strategies for the management of recurrent pyoderma. Proceedings of the Nineteenth World Small Animal Veterinary Association Congress, Durban, South Africa, 1994, pp 241–245.
4. DeBoer DJ: Management of chronic and recurrent pyoderma in the dog, in Bonagura JD (ed): *Kirk's Current Veterinary Therapy XII.* Philadelphia, WB Saunders, 1995, pp 611–617.
5. Scott DW, Miller WH, Griffin CE: *Muller & Kirk's Small Animal Dermatology,* ed 5. Philadelphia, WB Saunders, 1995, pp 279–328.
6. Mason IS, Lloyd DH: The role of allergy in the development of canine pyoderma. *J Small Anim Pract* 30:216–218, 1989.
7. Mason IS: Hypersensitivity and the multiplication of staphylococci on canine skin (PhD thesis). London, University of London, 1990, pp 1–172.
8. McEwan NA: Bacterial adherence to canine corneocytes, in Von Tscharner C, Halliwell REW (eds): *Advances in Veterinary Dermatology,* vol 1. London, Baillière Tindall, 1990, p 454.
9. Horwitz LN, Ihrke PJ: Canine seborrhea, in Kirk RW (ed): *Current Veterinary Therapy VI.* Philadelphia, WB Saunders, 1976, pp 519–524.
10. Ihrke PJ, Schwartzman RM, McGinley K, Horowitz L, Marples RR: Microbiology of normal and seborrheic canine skin. *Am J Vet Res* 39:1487–1489, 1978.
11. Kristensen S, Krogh HV: A study of skin diseases in dogs and cats—III. Microflora of the skin of dogs with chronic eczema. *Nord Vet Med* 30:223–230, 1978.
12. Fadok VA, Edwards MD: Advances in immunology. Proceedings of the Annual Meeting of the American Academy/College of Veterinary Dermatology (Resident Training Session Supplement), Santa Fe, New Mexico, 1995, pp 1–14.
13. Halliwell REW: Levels of IgE and IgG antibodies to staphylococcal antigens in normal dogs and in dogs with recurrent pyoderma. Proceedings American Academy/College of Veterinary Dermatology Annual Meeting, Phoenix, Arizona, 5, 1987.
14. Morales CA, Schultz KT, DeBoer DJ: Antistaphylococcal antibodies in dogs with recurrent staphylococcal pyoderma. *Vet Immmunol Immunopath* 42:137–147, 1994.
15. Ihrke PJ: Bacterial infections of the skin, in Greene CE (ed): *Infectious Diseases of the Dog and Cat.* Philadelphia, WB Saunders, 1990, pp 72–79.
16. Gross TL, Ihrke PJ, Walder EJ: *Veterinary Dermatopathology: A Macroscopic and Microscopic Evaluation of Canine and Feline Skin Disease.* St. Louis, Mosby–Year Book, 1992, pp 10–14, 238–240, 252–255.

Chapter 13

Management of Recurrent Pyoderma

Success or failure in the long-term management of recurrent pyoderma is contingent on multiple factors. These include the identification and appropriate management of underlying diseases, the commitment of the owner to identify recurrences, and the willingness of the owner to embark on multiple, sometimes complicated, therapeutic protocols. Complete therapeutic success is most likely to occur if underlying diseases are recognized and appropriately managed.[1-6] Recurrent pyoderma is termed *idiopathic* only after all attempts to identify underlying, predisposing factors have failed (see Chapter 12).

Extensive client communication and counseling are required because recurrent pyoderma commonly is a lifelong disease. An informed owner is much more likely to sustain the commitment required for successful long-term management. Owners should be told that unless a readily treatable underlying disease is identified, management usually requires long-term therapy for identified triggering underlying diseases, owner vigilance in recognizing early recurrence, lifelong shampoo therapy, long-term antibiotic manipulations, and possible immunomodulatory therapy (Table 13-1).

Prognosis may vary with age. Young dogs may occasionally outgrow the tendency to develop recurrent infections. Conversely, recurrent pyoderma that develops in older dogs indicates the possibility of diminished immune surveillance associated with underlying visceral disease such as occult neoplasia or pituitary-dependent hyperadrenocorticism.

There are no accepted guidelines with respect to how frequently pyoderma must occur for the clinician and owner to consider long-term continuous management versus simply treating each recurrence as a separate event. Owners should be instructed to keep a record of episodes of infection. In general, if pyoderma recurs only three or four times annually, it probably is more economical and reasonable to treat each event separately. Alternatively, contingent on circumstances and the wishes of the owner, weekly antibacterial shampoo therapy could be instituted to ascertain whether this regimen alone could diminish the frequency of infection. If owners are willing and able to shampoo their dogs frequently and shampoo alone diminishes the frequency of recurrence, this option is always available. However, this decision should be made jointly by the owner and clinician in each case.

MANAGEMENT OF UNDERLYING DISEASES AND OTHER CONTRIBUTING FACTORS

If underlying diseases are identified, curative therapy for the predisposing disease may completely prevent recurrences of secondary pyoderma. For example, successful long-term thyroid hormone replacement therapy in a hypothyroid dog may completely prevent recurrences of pyoderma. Continuous prophylactic flea control may be required of the owner for the long-term prevention of recurrent pyoderma in a dog that develops bacterial skin disease secondary to flea allergy dermatitis. Many of the skin diseases that act as triggers for recurrent pyoderma can be controlled but not cured and require continuous

TABLE 13-1
CONSIDERATIONS FOR SUCCESSFUL MANAGEMENT OF RECURRENT PYODERMA

- Long-term therapy for identified triggering underlying diseases
- Owner vigilance in recognizing early recurrence
- Lifelong shampoo therapy
- Possible immunomodulatory therapy
- Long-term antibiotic manipulations

management decisions by the clinician and the owner. Dogs with atopic dermatitis and defects in cornification rarely respond completely to appropriate therapy and instead require lifelong maintenance and owner commitment.

Long-term topical antibacterial shampoos, immunomodulatory therapy, and extended regimens of antibiotics should be considered sequentially in the management of recurrent pyoderma if a search for underlying causes has not led to a predisposing disease that can be managed successfully. These therapeutic options should be initiated only after appropriate antibiotic and adjunctive therapy has completely ameliorated the last recurrence of infection (see Chapter 10).

Frequent topical antibacterial shampoo therapy should be used initially in an attempt to diminish the frequency of recurrent infection. If beneficial in reducing recurrences, antibacterial shampoo therapy can be continued indefinitely. Adjunctive immunomodulatory therapy, either bacterin preparations or nonbacterial immunostimulants, may be attempted in dogs with confirmed or suspected defects of the immune system, dogs with identified but incompletely managed underlying diseases, and in dogs with idiopathic recurrent pyoderma. Extended regimens of antibiotics usually are given at dosages considered to be subtherapeutic. Consequently, they should be considered as a last resort after shampoo and immunomodulatory therapy have failed to prevent frequent recurrences.

TOPICAL ANTIBACTERIAL THERAPY

Antibacterial shampoos containing either benzoyl peroxide, benzoyl peroxide and sulfur, chlorhexidine, triclosan, or ethyl lactate are useful in the management of canine pyoderma (see Chapter 10). An ideal topical product for use in recurrent pyoderma should both aid in the initial resolution of the infection and assist in the prevention of relapses by limiting the bacterial surface flora. Benzoyl peroxide is particularly attractive as an active agent because it exhibits follicular flushing, degreasing, and keratolytic activity, as well as antibacterial efficacy. Because most recurrent canine pyodermas involve hair follicles, follicular flushing would be expected to aid in preventing recrudescence. Early work by Lloyd and Reyss-Brion indicates that benzoyl peroxide may diminish the frequency of occurrence of canine pyoderma in dogs with recurrent disease.[7] Kwochka and Kowalski have shown that benzoyl peroxide has superior prophylactic activity against *Staphylococcus intermedius* in comparison to chlorhexidine, povidone–iodine, and triclosan.[8] Although many current products are effective and cosmetically acceptable, the author's current shampoo of choice for recurrent pyoderma contains both benzoyl peroxide and sulfur. Benzoyl peroxide–containing shampoos still may be drying and irritating with long-term use, although the better, currently available products containing benzoyl peroxide are less drying than those available a decade ago. If a frequent (two or three times weekly) regimen of shampooing with benzoyl peroxide is not well tolerated, the clinician can either switch to a less drying and potentially less irritating active ingredient or use a moisturizing rinse. Other beneficial active ingredients that may be less drying include ethyl lactate and chlorhexidine.

Antibacterial shampoos should be used at least weekly and preferably twice weekly in an attempt to diminish the frequency of recurrent pyoderma. This requires either a substantial time commitment from the owner or the financial commitment of arranging to have it done elsewhere.

Antibacterial shampoos used as a sole method of diminishing the frequency or preventing the recurrence of pyoderma have been most beneficial in the management of superficial spreading pyoderma and superficial folliculitis. Shampoo therapy rarely is successful as the sole method for preventing the recurrence of deep pyoderma; however, it may be beneficial in deep pyoderma as an adjunct to immunomodulatory and extended-regimen antibiotic therapy.

IMMUNOMODULATORY THERAPY

Immunomodulatory therapy remains controversial in veterinary dermatology.[1–6,9,10] Available products consist of either killed bacterial products for injection or oral drugs

> If underlying diseases are identified, curative therapy for the predisposing disease may completely prevent recurrences of secondary pyoderma.

that may alter lymphocyte function (see Chapter 10). Most evaluations have been highly subjective because immunomodulatory therapy usually is used in conjunction with topical antibacterial therapy and systemic antibiotics.

A well-controlled, double-blind placebo-controlled study by DeBoer and others indicated efficacy in 40% of recurrent pyoderma beyond placebo effect for a product consisting of bacterial antigen made from human strains of *Staphylococcus aureus*, serotypes I and III.[11] Staphage Lysate (SPL)® (Delmont Laboratories) is injected subcutaneously at a dosage of 0.5 ml twice weekly or 1 ml weekly. Because the product is packaged in 10-ml vials, at least two vials (20 weeks) should be used to determine any efficacy. Successful usage, as determined by a decrease in either frequency or severity of infection, usually indicates the need for lifelong therapy. Currently, this product is the most commonly employed immunomodulatory product used for the management of recurrent canine pyoderma.[2-6,9,10]

Autogenous bacterins prepared directly from organisms isolated from the affected dog have only limited use. Because adverse reactions to autogenous bacterins are relatively common, they are generally used either after treatment failure with Staphage Lysate (SPL)® or in countries where suitable commercially prepared products are not available.

Levamisole, a levoisomer of tetramisole sold as a vermifuge, probably is the most commonly employed nonbacterial immunomodulatory drug used for the management of recurrent pyoderma. Evidence indicates that levamisole may alter lymphocyte and phagocyte immune function. The drug reputedly has a "window" effect, whereby dosages too high or too low may cause immunosuppression rather than immunostimulation. The recommended dosage is 2.2 mg/kg PO given every other day. Controlled studies have not been performed. Many dermatologists indicate anecdotally that they have seen some efficacy in isolated cases; however, it is probably less than 20%. The author considers levamisole as a "last resort" after other therapy has been unsuccessful.

Cimetidine, an H_2 histamine receptor blocker, theoretically may reduce immunosuppression by modulating cytokine production. Twice-daily doses of 3 to 4 mg/kg PO have been suggested. Cimetidine seems to be safe in the dog but is quite expensive. Controlled studies have not been performed, and efficacy data are not available.

EXTENDED REGIMENS OF ANTIBIOTIC THERAPY

Extended regimens of systemic antibiotics frequently maintain remission in dogs with recurrent pyoderma (Table 13-2). Full dosages may be implemented long-term, but this option is used infrequently. Antibiotic dosages conventionally considered to be subtherapeutic are utilized more commonly to control cost and diminish the frequency of administration. Extended antibiotic regimens using subtherapeutic dosages should be considered as a last resort. This modality of therapy should be reserved for circumstances where underlying causes either cannot be identified or cannot be managed successfully. If feasible, long-term shampoo and immunomodulatory therapy should be attempted before extended regimens of antibiotics are considered.

Substantial drawbacks are associated with the extended administration of systemic antibiotics at subtherapeutic doses. Potential risks include undesirable effects in the patient, induction of antibiotic resistance, and the formation and possible dissemination of resistant strains of bacteria in the environment. Relatively high cost is an additional drawback of long-term antibiotic therapy using any regimen.

Risks to the patient include the potential for systemic or cutaneous adverse drug reactions. Vomiting or diarrhea may be seen as a sequela to either changes in the gastrointestinal flora or direct irritation of the gastrointestinal tract. Although unlikely, severe hypersensitivity reactions including life-threatening anaphylaxis may be seen with extended use of systemic antibiotics. Likewise, cutaneous adverse drug reactions also may occur with extended usage. Skin reactions can vary from trivial eruptions to rare syndromes that may be potentially life-threatening, such as

> An ideal topical product for use in recurrent pyoderma should both aid in the initial resolution of the infection and assist in the prevention of relapses by limiting the bacterial surface flora.

TABLE 13-2
EXTENDED ANTIBIOTIC THERAPY FOR RECURRENT PYODERMA

- **PREFERRED ANTIBIOTICS**
  Cephalexin
  Oxacillin
  Clavulanic acid–potentiated amoxicillin
  Enrofloxacin

- **DOSING OPTIONS**
  Every other week (full daily dose)*
  2 days per week (full daily dose)
  Once a day
  Every other day

*Author's personal preference.

---

erythema multiforme major and toxic epidermal necrolysis.

Antibiotic-resistant populations of bacteria occur as the result of antibiotic usage. Subtherapeutic antibiotic dosages commonly employed in the long-term management of recurrent pyoderma increase the likelihood that resistant bacterial populations will emerge through the exertion of selection pressure on bacterial populations. Multiple repercussions may occur. From the narrow perspective of the owner and clinician managing an individual case, antibiotic resistance diminishes the potential choice of antibiotics available to successfully manage bacterial infection. From a global perspective, indiscriminate use of antibiotics may lead to the increased frequency of infections from highly resistant pathogens that may defy currently available treatments. All health care professionals have the moral responsibility to use antibiotics in a manner to decrease the likelihood that more antibiotic-resistant bacterial strains will emerge.

It should be emphasized again that extended regimens should not be used until the pyoderma has been brought under complete control by a standard course of appropriate antibiotic therapy (see Chapter 10). In general, antibiotics such as penicillin, ampicillin, amoxicillin, tetracycline, and nonpotentiated sulfonamides considered to be poor choices for the management of canine pyoderma obviously are even less effective choices for the management of recurrent pyoderma. In addition, antibiotics such as erythromycin and lincomycin, where resistance develops rapidly with use, also are poor choices for extended regimens in recurrent infection.

The potential for keratoconjunctivitis sicca plus perceived diminished efficacy with long-term administration also precludes the use of trimethoprim-potentiated sulfonamides for extended regimens. To the author's knowledge, there are no reports documenting use of ormetoprim-potentiated sulfonamides for long-term therapy.

Antibiotics used most commonly for extended regimens with minimal side effects and minimal induced bacterial resistance include the first-generation cephalosporin **cephalexin** and the β-lactamase–resistant synthetic penicillin **oxacillin**.[3-6,9] **Clavulanic acid–potentiated amoxicillin** also has been employed in extended regimens.[6,9] **Enrofloxacin** is an additional attractive choice in chronic cases complicated by bacterial resistance or mixed infection.[6,9]

The author's first choice in most cases of recurrent pyoderma that require extended antibiotic regimens given in subtherapeutic dosages is cephalexin. Oxacillin, enrofloxacin, and clavulanic acid–potentiated amoxicillin usually are reserved for patients that do not respond to cephalexin. Enrofloxacin may be the best choice for extended-regimen therapy in deep, recurrent pyoderma complicated by impaired drainage routes and sequestered foci of infection.

Many different regimens for long-term, extended antibiotic usage have been recommended.[2-6,9] Popular options include dosing every other week, 2 days per week at full daily dose, once a day, or every other day. Options such as every-other-week therapy and 2-days-per-week therapy have been termed *pulse therapy* because full therapeutic doses are given on an intermittent basis.

In every-other-week dosing, 1 week of medication (at the full, recommended daily dose) is followed by 1 week "off medication." If this regimen prevents recurrence, the clinician and owner can consider extending the duration of "time off" antibiotics in gradual increments (e.g., 2 weeks, 3 weeks). The author has not attempted to increase the

> Extended regimens of systemic antibiotics frequently maintain remission in dogs with recurrent pyoderma.

"off time" to greater than 3 weeks. According to DeBoer, most recurrent pyoderma will recrudesce if "off times" greater than 3 weeks are attempted.[5]

Two-days-per-week dosing at full daily dosage is an additional popular regimen. Although compliance may be difficult to achieve with all intermittent regimens, clients have indicated that 2-days-per-week dosing is more difficult to remember correctly than every-other-week dosing.

Theoretically, once-a-day and every-other-day dosing are more likely to induce resistance. However, clinical experience has not shown a difference in induced resistance with any of the regimens mentioned above. Kwochka recently summarized research data indicating that suboptimal therapy may cause "structural alterations in the bacteria, enhanced phagocytosis, increased bactericidal activity of serum, decreased ability to adhere to corneocytes, and alterations in enzyme systems."[3] These beneficial effects may explain the surprising efficacy of suboptimal dosages used for extended regimens; however, extended regimens should always be used as a last resort, and therapy should be monitored carefully.

REFERENCES

1. DeBoer DJ: Strategies for management of recurrent pyoderma in dogs, in DeBoer DJ (ed): *Veterinary Clinics of North America: Advances in Clinical Dermatology.* Philadelphia, WB Saunders, 1990, pp 1509–1524.
2. Ihrke PJ: Bacterial infections of the skin, in Greene CE (ed): *Infectious Diseases of the Dog and Cat.* Philadelphia, WB Saunders, 1990, pp 72–79.
3. Kwochka KW: Recurrent pyoderma, in Griffin CE, Kwochka KW, MacDonald JM (eds): *Current Veterinary Dermatology.* St. Louis, Mosby–Year Book, 1993, pp 3–21.
4. Ihrke PJ: Antibiotic therapy and strategies for the management of recurrent pyoderma. Proceedings of the Nineteenth World Small Animal Veterinary Association Congress, Durban, South Africa, 1994, pp 241–245.
5. DeBoer DJ: Management of chronic and recurrent pyoderma in the dog, in Bonagura JD (ed): *Kirk's Current Veterinary Therapy XII.* Philadelphia, WB Saunders, 1995, pp 611–617.
6. Scott DW, Miller WH, Griffin CE: *Muller & Kirk's Small Animal Dermatology,* ed 5. Philadelphia, WB Saunders, 1995, pp 218–221, 279–328.
7. Lloyd DH, Reyss-Brion A: Le peroxide de benzoyle: Efficacite clinique et bacteriologique dans le traitement des pyodermites chroniques. *Prat Med Chirurg Anim Compag* 19:445–448, 1984.
8. Kwochka KW, Kowalski JJ: Prophylactic efficacy of four antibacterial shampoos against *Staphylococcus intermedius* in dogs. *Am J Vet Res* 52:115–118, 1991.
9. Mason I, Moriello K: Management of infectious disorders, in Moriello K, Mason I (eds): *Handbook of Small Animal Dermatology.* Oxford, Pergamon, 1995, pp 287–294.
10. Lloyd DH: Therapy for canine pyoderma, in Kirk RW, Bonagura JD (eds): *Current Veterinary Therapy XI.* Philadelphia, WB Saunders, 1992, pp 539–544.
11. DeBoer DJ, Moriello KA, Thomes CB, et al: Evaluation of a commercial staphylococcal bacterin for management of idiopathic recurrent superficial pyoderma in dogs. *Am J Vet Res* 51:636–639, 1990.

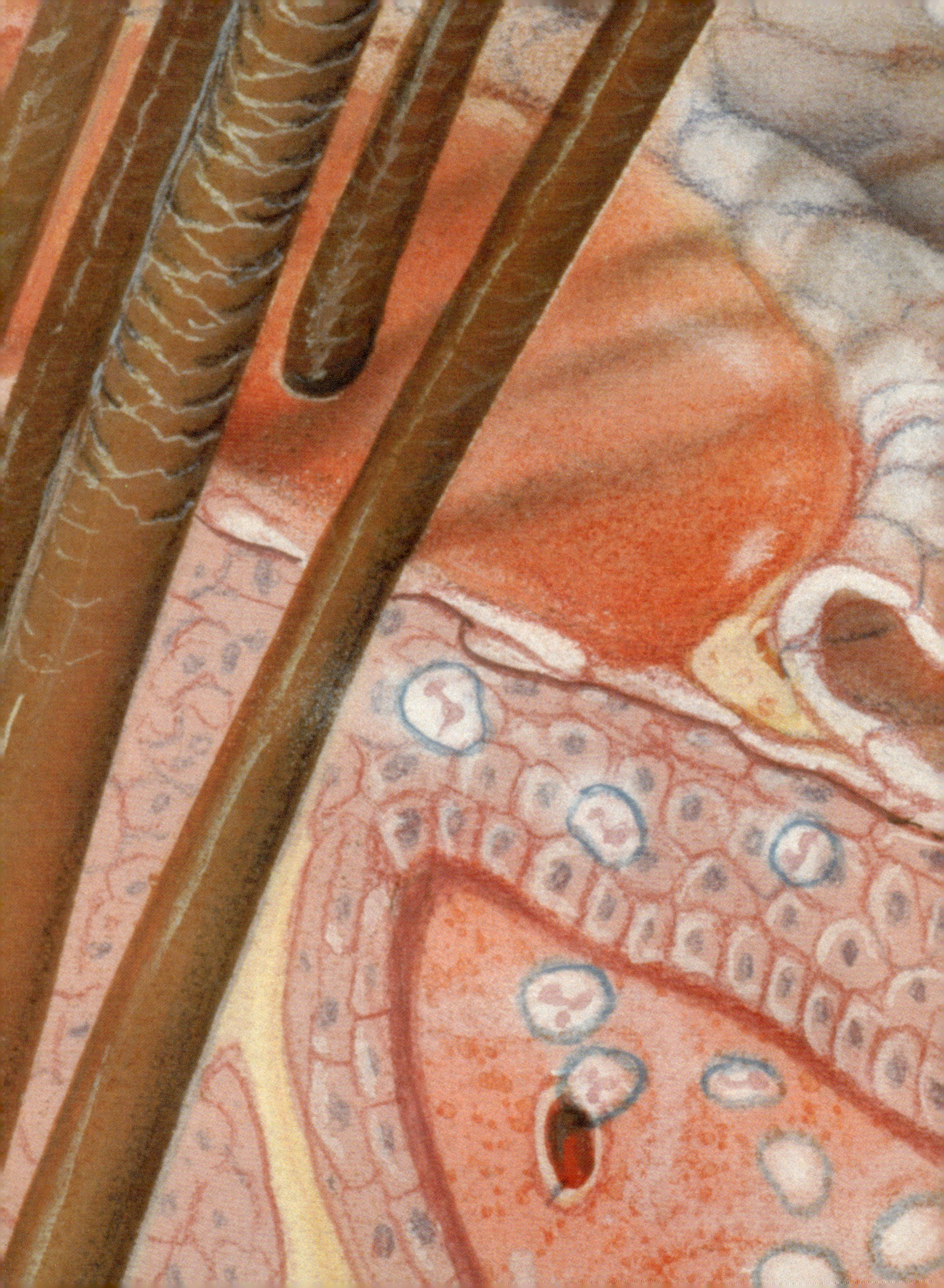

Chapter 14

Future Developments

GENERAL CONSIDERATIONS

Single episodes of canine pyoderma usually can be managed adequately with therapeutic regimens currently available (see Chapters 6–8 and 10). However, recurrent infections still frequently defy attempts at identifying underlying triggering diseases or other predisposing causes. If underlying, predisposing factors cannot be identified in cases of recurrent canine pyoderma, recurrence remains the rule rather than the exception (see Chapter 12). New, more specific testing procedures for the evaluation of host immunocompetency in response to bacterial skin disease are needed (see Chapters 3 and 9). Manipulation of microbial flora and modification of the host response to pathogenic bacteria also may offer future advances in the prevention or management of recurrent staphylococcal skin infections. New systemic and topical antibacterial products may offer a greater range of efficacy and safety and improve our ability to cope with canine bacterial skin disease.

EVALUATION FOR IMMUNOCOMPETENCY

Fadok recently offered a "wish list" of techniques for potential use in the evaluation of canine pyoderma.[1,2] These techniques include:

- Assessment of T and B lymphocyte response to specific bacterial antigens and super-antigens rather than plant-derived mitogens
- Assessment of T cell phenotypes in both skin and blood
- Identification of specific staphylococcal strains by genetic markers
- White blood cell function tests (for neutrophils, lymphocytes, and macrophages)
- Assessment of bacterial super-antigen effects in dogs[1,2]

In the past, measurement of antibody response has been the primary method of assaying immune competence and susceptibility to disease. The methodology required to assay cell-mediated immunity is substantially more complicated and fraught with potential laboratory error and misinterpretation.[3] Antigen-specific cell-mediated immunity can be measured by the following assays: delayed-type hypersensitivity, leukocyte migration inhibition, adoptive transfer, leukocyte proliferation, cytokine release, and cytotoxicity.[3]

Leukocyte migration inhibition, lymphocyte proliferation, cytokine release, and cytotoxicity assays seem to be the most applicable for the study of the immunologic response to staphylococcal antigens.[3,4] Lymphocyte proliferation assays utilizing specific bacterial antigens and super-antigens may provide more useful information.[1,2] Currently, cytokine release assays are performed most commonly by utilizing indirect bioassays. However, assays directly measuring cytokine release offer better hope for more specific determinations.[3,5] As species-specific reagents for cytokines become available, it may be possible to directly measure cytokine release in response to staphylococcal antigens. Cytotoxicity assays have the advantage of offering measurement of effector function.[3] These assays could prove particularly useful in assessing the immune response to bacterial skin disease.

MANIPULATION OF MICROBIAL FLORA

The establishment of resident nonvir-

> Manipulation of microbial flora and modification of the host response to pathogenic bacteria may offer future advances in the prevention or management of recurrent staphylococcal skin infections.

ulent strains of *Staphylococcus* in an attempt to prevent pathogenic bacteria from colonizing the skin and inducing infection has long been a goal of microbiologists and dermatologists.[6-9] If nonvirulent strains competitively bind to specific cell surface receptors, infection could theoretically be prevented.[10] However, attempts at maintaining resident nonvirulent bacterial strains have yielded mixed results.[9,11,12] Staphylococcal flora are established gradually in puppies after birth.[13] Allaker and others have suggested the possibility of substituting a bacterial antagonist to prevent colonization by virulent strains of *Staphylococcus intermedius* in dogs at increased risk for the development of pyoderma.[13,14]

The process of bacterial colonization of the skin involves irreversible adherence via a bacterial adhesion that is attracted to specific skin receptors.[10] Teichoic acids are important staphylococcal adhesins that binds to fibronectin.[10,15] Darmstadt and Lane speculate that the "topical application of a purified bacterial adhesion such as teichoic acid or of cell surface receptors such as fibronectin, might competitively block pathogenic staphylococci and streptococci from adhering to the skin."[10]

Fadok further speculates about the creation of a mutation in the staphylococcal genome to create a bacterium with less virulence but more adherence to skin surface receptors.[2] This modified *Staphylococcus* could compete with pathogenic strains. In addition, it might be possible to create a lytic virus with the capacity to kill canine *S. intermedius* and thus treat canine pyoderma. It also is intriguing to speculate that a topical product could be developed to alter the surface ecosystem microenvironment such that *S. intermedius* overgrowth is prevented.[2]

MODIFICATION OF HOST RESPONSE

Immunologic response to bacterial infections theoretically could be altered in a variety of ways to aid in host immune targeting of *S. intermedius* and discourage recurrence of infection. In addition, the immune response conceivably could be altered in dogs with inappropriately severe inflammatory responses to staphylococci.

> Bacterial super-antigens may play a role in the severe inflammation evident in some cases of canine pyoderma. Topical or systemic products could be developed that modify host response.

New methods of stimulating cell-mediated response or antibody production in dogs in the face of a *S. intermedius* challenge could be useful both as a therapeutic measure and as a way to prevent or reduce the severity of future infections with this pathogen. According to DeBoer, a *S. intermedius* lysate is under development.[16] A canine *Staphylococcus*-based product would have the theoretical advantage of containing bacterial antigens specific for canine skin infections. However, such a product might contain less protein A, a potentially important immune response–inducing antigen present in higher concentration in lysates from human source *Staphylococcus aureus*.

Methods of antigen delivery designed to produce maximum stimulation of cell-mediated immunity have been an area of recent research interest.[3] Newer synthetic antigen delivery systems include antigen complexing with biodegradable microspheres (liposomes), and immunostimulating complexes (ISCOMs) have been developed.[17-20] The use of these newer methodologies theoretically could diminish the frequency of administration currently required for *Staphylococcus*-based bacterin products.

Bacterial super-antigens may play a role in the severe inflammation evident in some cases of canine pyoderma.[21] Topical or systemic products could be developed that either promote faulty white cell function or deplete specific T lymphocyte subsets that respond to staphylococcal super-antigens.[2]

NEW ANTIBACTERIAL PRODUCTS

New products constantly are being developed for both veterinary and human medicine. Although many antibiotics are useful in the management of canine pyoderma, the ideal antibiotic still has not been developed. Theoretically, the ideal antibiotic would have the beneficial properties of concentrating in the skin, a long duration of activity, a narrow spectrum of activity directed against *S. intermedius*, no potential for the development of bacterial resistance, and no deleterious side effects as well as being inexpensive! An ideal topical antibacterial agent for use either in a shampoo base or as a final rinse would have similar properties.

REFERENCES

1. Fadok VA: Immunologic testing for the practitioner: Autoimmune diseases and immunodeficiency. Proceedings of the George H. Muller Stanford Veterinary Dermatology Seminar, 11, 1993.
2. Fadok VA: Future directions: Diagnostics and therapy for the 21st century. Proceedings of the George H. Muller Stanford Veterinary Dermatology Seminar, 11, 1993.
3. Coe Clough NE, Roth JA: Methods for assessing cell-mediated immunity in infectious disease resistance and in the development of vaccines. JAVMA 206:1208–1216, 1995.
4. Abbas AK, Lichtman AH, Pober JS: *Cellular and Molecular Immunology*, ed 2. Philadelphia, WB Saunders, 1994, pp 320–336.
5. Mossman TR, Fong TAT: Specific assays for cytokine production by T cells. *J Immunol Methods* 116:151–158, 1989.
6. Aly R, Shinefield HR, Maibach HI: *Staphylococcus aureus* adherence to nasal epithelial cell: Studies of some parameters, in Maibach H, Aly R (eds): *Skin Microbiology: Relevance to Clinical Infection*. New York, Springer-Verlag, 1981, pp 171–179.
7. Feingold DS: Bacterial adherence, colonization and pathogenicity. *Arch Dermatol* 122:161–163, 1986.
8. Roth RR, James WD: Microbiology of the skin: Resident flora, ecology, infection. *J Am Acad Dermatol* 30:367–390, 1989.
9. Allaker RP, Noble WC: Microbial interactions on skin, in Noble WC (ed): *The Skin Microflora and Microbial Skin Disease*. Cambridge, Cambridge University Press, 1993, pp 331–354.
10. Darmstadt GL, Lane AT: Impetigo: An overview. *Pediatr Dermatol* 11(4):293–303, 1994.
11. Shienfield HR, Ribble JC, Boris M, et al: Bacterial interference: Its effect on nursery acquired infection with *Staphylococcus aureus* I: Preliminary observations on artificial colonization of newborns. *Am J Dis Child* 105:646–654, 1963.
12. Steele RW: Recurrent staphylococcal infection in families. *Arch Dermatol* 116:189–190, 1980.
13. Allaker RP, Jensen L, Lloyd DH, Lamport AI: Colonization of neonatal puppies by staphylococci. *Br Vet J* 148:523–528, 1992.
14. Allaker RP, Lloyd DH, Bailey RM: Population sizes and frequency of staphylococci at mucocutaneous sites on healthy dogs. *Vet Rec* 130:303–304, 1992.
15. Kuusela P, Vartio T, Vuento M, et al: Binding sites of streptococci and staphylococci in fibronectin. *Infect Immun* 45:433–436, 1984.
16. DeBoer DJ: Management of chronic and recurrent pyoderma in the dog, in Bonagura JD (ed): *Kirk's Current Veterinary Therapy XII*. Philadelphia, WB Saunders, 1995, pp 611–617.
17. Eldridge JH, Staas JK, Meulbroek JA, et al: Biodegradable microspheres as a vaccine delivery system. *Mol Immunol* 28:287–294, 1991.
18. Gregoriadis G: Immunological adjuvants: A role for liposomes. *Immunol Today* 11:89–97, 1990.
19. Lovgren K, Morein B: The ISCOM: An antigen delivery system with built-in adjuvant. *Mol Immunol* 28:285–286, 1991.
20. Mowat AM, Donachie AM: ISCOMs: A novel strategy for mucosal immunization? *Immunol Today* 12:383–385, 1991.
21. Fadok VA, Edwards MD: Advances in immunology. Proceedings of the Annual Meeting of the American Academy/College of Veterinary Dermatology (Resident Training Session Supplement), Santa Fe, New Mexico, 1995, pp 1–14.

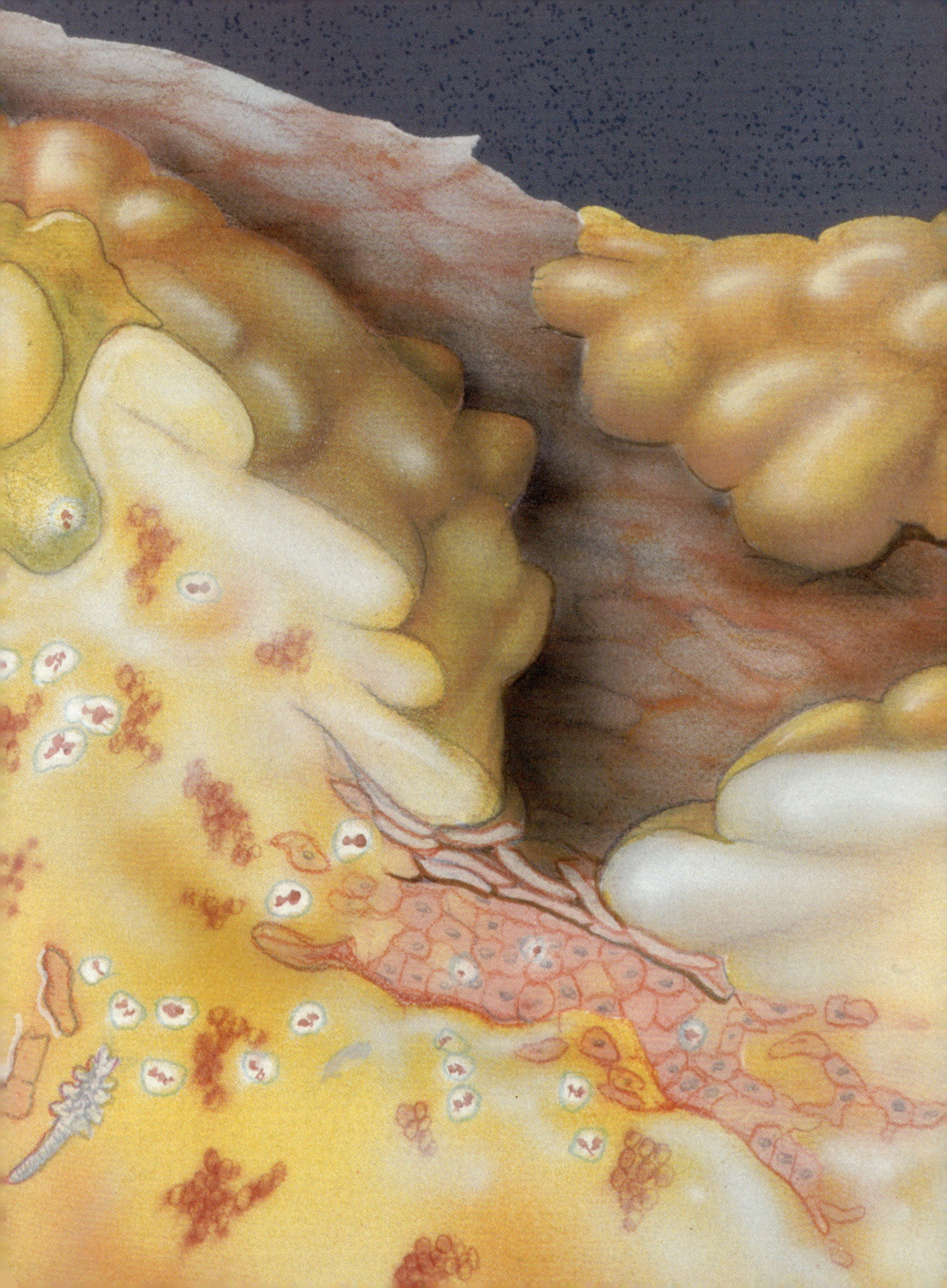

Index

Note: i refers to illustrations; t refers to tables.

A

Acne, canine, 16t, 20, 46–47
Allergy
　and recurrent canine pyoderma, 78, 78t
Alopecia, 19
Aminoglycosides, 66–67
Amoxicillin, 65–66
Amoxicillin, clavulanic acid–potentiated, 64t, 66–69, 86, 86t
Ampicillin, 65–66
Antibacterial agents, *see also* Antibiotic therapy
Antibiotic sensitivity
　bacterial culture and identification and, 61
Antibiotic therapy, *see also specific drugs*
　new products, 90
　systemic, 63–69
　　basic principles, 63t
　　clinical trials, 66
　　culture and sensitivity studies, 65–66
　　extended regimens for recurrent pyoderma, 85–87, 86t
　　rational selection, 66–69
　　useful oral antibiotics, 64t, 67t
　topical, 69–71
　　gels, creams, and ointments, 71
　　shampoos, 69–70, 84
　　soaks and whirlpools, 70–71
Atopic dermatitis
　and recurrent canine pyoderma, 78, 78t

B

Bacteria
　normal, of canine skin and hair, 3–4
Bacterial culture
　and antibiotic sensitivity, 61
　and identification, 61
Bacterial folliculitis
　deep, and furunculosis, 41–46, 42i, 45t
　superficial, 20, 30–35, 31i
Bacterial hypersensitivity, 79, 79t
Bacterial infection
　anatomy of canine skin and, 3
　classification based on depth of, 15
　host factors and susceptibility to, 2t

Bacterins
　in immunomodulatory therapy, 72, 85
Benzoyl peroxide, 72, 85
　and sulfur, 70, 84
Biopsy, skin
　in canine pyoderma, 58–61
　　indications, 59
　　method selection, 59
　　preparation for submission, 61
　　technique, 59–61
　　timing and lesion selection, 59
Bullae, hemorrhagic, 20
Bullous impetigo
　and recurrent canine pyoderma, 81, 81t

C

Callus pyoderma, 16t, 20, 51–53
Cefadroxil, 64t, 66–67, 67t, 68–69
Cellulitis, 16t, 53–56, 54i
Cephalexin, 64t, 65–67, 67t, 68–69, 86, 86t
Cephalothin, 65
Cheyletiellosis
　and recurrent canine pyoderma, 78, 78t
Chloramphenicol, 66, 67
Chlorhexidine, 70, 84
Cimetidine, 73, 85
Ciprofloxacin, 67
Classification, of canine pyoderma, 15–17
　deep, 15t, 16t, 17
　superficial, 15t, 16t, 17
　surface, 15–16, 15t, 16t
Clavulanic acid–potentiated amoxicillin *see Amoxicillin.*
Clindamycin, 66–68
Clinical signs, of canine pyoderma
　general, 19–20
　　distribution of lesions, 20
　　primary skin lesions, 19
　　secondary skin lesions, 19–20
Cloxacillin, 66
Collarettes, 19, 35, 36i, 37–38
Cornification, diseases of
　and recurrent canine pyoderma, 78t, 79
Creams, antibacterial, 71
Culture, bacterial
　and antibiotic sensitivity, 61
　and identification, 61
Cytology
　in canine pyoderma, 58, 58t

D

Deep bacterial folliculitis and furunculosis, 16t, 41–46, 42i
Deep pyoderma, 41–56
    bacterial folliculitis and furunculosis, 16t, 41–46, 42i
    callus pyoderma, 51–52
    canine acne, 16t, 46–47
    cellulitis, 16t, 53–56, 54i
    classification, 15t, 16t, 17
    differential diagnosis, 16t
    German shepherd dog pyoderma, 16t, 52–53
    muzzle folliculitis and furunculosis, 16t, 46–47
    pedal folliculitis and furunculosis, 16t, 49–51
    pressure-point pyoderma, 51–52
    pyotraumatic folliculitis, 16t, 47–49
    recurrent, 81–82
Demodicosis
    and recurrent canine pyoderma, 78–79, 78t
Dermatitis
    pyotraumatic, 16t, 20, 21–22, 80, 80t
Dermatophytosis
    and recurrent canine pyoderma, 78t, 79
Diagnosis, of canine pyoderma
    diagnostic procedures, 57–62
        bacterial culture, 61
        cytologic examination, 58
        evaluation for immunocompetency, 61–62
        general considerations, 57
        skin biopsy, 58–61
        skin scrapings, 57–58
    differential, 16t

E

Endocrine diseases
    and recurrent canine pyoderma, 78t, 79
Enrofloxacin, 64t, 65–69, 67t, 86, 86t
Epidermis, canine
    as barrier against bacterial infection, 3, 5i
Erythromycin, 64t, 65–67, 67t
Ethyl lactate, 70, 84
Etiology
    of canine pyoderma, 3–6
Excoriations, 19

F

Facial-fold intertrigo, 16t, 22–25

Flea allergy dermatitis
    and recurrent canine pyoderma, 78, 78t
Fluoroquinolones, 66, 68–69, *see also Enrofloxacin*
Folliculitis
    deep bacterial, and furunculosis, 16t, 20, 41–46, 42i, 45t
    muzzle, and furunculosis, 16t, 46–47
    pedal, and furunculosis, 16t, 49–51
    pyotraumatic, 16t, 47–49
    superficial bacterial, 20, 30–35, 31i
Food allergy
    and recurrent canine pyoderma, 78, 78t
Furunculosis
    deep bacterial folliculitis and, 16t, 41–46, 42i, 45t
    muzzle folliculitis and, 16t, 46–47
    pedal folliculitis and, 16t, 49–51

G

Gels, antibacterial, 71
Genodermatoses
    and recurrent canine pyoderma, 78t, 79
German shepherd dog pyoderma, 16t, 52–53
Glucocorticoids
    and recurrent canine pyoderma, 78

H

Hair, canine
    normal microflora of, 3–6
Host response, to infection, 10–12, 11i
    beneficial, 10
    deleterious, 12
    modification of, 90
Hot spots, 16t, 21–22
Hyperadrenocorticism, pituitary-dependent
    and recurrent canine pyoderma, 78t, 79
Hyperglucocorticoidism, iatrogenic
    and recurrent canine pyoderma, 78t, 79
Hypersensitivity, bacterial
    and recurrent canine pyoderma, 79, 79t
Hypothyroidism
    and recurrent canine pyoderma, 78t, 79

I

Idiopathic recurrent pyoderma, 82

Immunocompetency
    evaluation for, 61–62
        future developments in, 89
Immunodeficiency
    and recurrent canine pyoderma, 78t, 79–80
Immunomodulatory therapy
    for canine pyoderma, 71–73
        bacterin preparations, 72
        nonbacterial immunostimulants, 72–73
    for recurrent canine pyoderma, 84–85
Immunostimulants, nonbacterial
    in immunomodulatory therapy, 72–73
Impetigo, 16t, 20, 27–30, 28i
Infection
    bacterial, anatomy of canine skin and, 3
    host response to, 10–12
    susceptibility to, 9–10, 9t
Inflammation, 10, 11i
    of hair follicles, recurrent pyoderma and, 78t, 79
Intertrigo, 16t, 20, 22–25, 80–81, 80t

K

Keratinization defects, primary
    and recurrent canine pyoderma, 78t

L

Levamisole, 72–73, 85
Lincomycin, 64t, 65–67, 67t
Lip-fold intertrigo, 16t, 22–25

M

Malassezia dermatitis
    and recurrent canine pyoderma, 78t, 79
Management, of canine pyoderma
    complicating factors in, 75–76
        coexisting problems, 76t
        external factors, 76
        inappropriate initial therapy, 75
        sequestered foci of infection, 75–76
    future developments in, 89–91
    overview of, 63–74, 63t
        assessment of therapy, 73
        general considerations, 63
        immunomodulatory therapy, 71–73

        initial management, 73
        systemic antibiotic therapy, 63–69, 64t, 67t
        topical antibacterial therapy, 69–71
    recurrent pyoderma, 83–87, 83t
        extended antibiotic regimens, 85–87, 86t
        immunomodulatory therapy, 71–73
        topical antibiotic therapy, 84
        underlying diseases, 83–84
Microflora
    alterations of in skin disease, 6–7
    manipulation of, 89–90
    normal, canine skin and hair, 3–6
Moist dermatitis, acute, 16t, 21–22
Mucocutaneous pyoderma, 16t, 20, 25–26, 80t, 81
Mupirocin, 71
Muzzle folliculitis and furunculosis, 66t, 46–47

N

Neoplasia, occult
    and recurrent canine pyoderma, 78t, 79
Nodules, 19
Nonstaphylococcal pyoderma, 79t, 80

O

Obesity-fold intertrigo, 16t, 22–25
Occult neoplasia
    and recurrent canine neoplasia, 78t, 79
Ointments, antibacterial, 71
Oral antibiotics
    for canine pyoderma management, 64t, 67t
Ormetoprim-potentiated sulfonamides, 64t, 65–67, 67t
    sulfadiazine, 67
    sulfadimethoxine, 67–68
Oxacillin, 64t, 65–67, 67t, 68–69, 86, 86t

P

Papules, 19
Parasitic diseases, allergic
    and recurrent canine pyoderma, 78–79, 78t
Pathogenesis
    of canine pyoderma, 3–5
Pathogens
    canine cutaneous, 6
    zoonotic potential of, 7
Pedal folliculitis and furunculosis, 16t, 49–51

Penicillin, 65–66
Pododermatitis, 49–51
Povidone-iodine, 70
Pressure-point pyoderma, 16t, 51–52
Primary skin lesions
　general clinical findings, 19
Puppy pyoderma, 16t, 27–30
Pustules, 19
Pyoderma, canine
　callus, 16t, 20, 51–53
　classification, 15–17
　　deep, 15t, 16t, 17
　　superficial, 15t, 16t, 17
　　surface, 15–16, 15t, 16t
　clinical findings, general, 19–20
　　distribution of lesions, 20
　　primary skin lesions, 19
　　secondary skin lesions, 19–20
　deep, 41–56
　　bacterial folliculitis and furunculosis, 41–46, 42i
　　callus pyoderma, 51–52
　　canine acne, 46–47
　　cellulitis, 53–56
　　German shepherd dog pyoderma, 16t, 52–53
　　muzzle folliculitis and furunculosis, 46–47
　　pedal folliculitis and furunculosis, 49–51
　　pressure-point pyoderma, 51–52
　　pyotraumatic folliculitis, 47–49
　diagnostic procedures, 57–62
　　bacterial culture, 61
　　cytologic examination, 58
　　evaluation for immunocompetency, 61–62
　　general considerations, 57
　　skin biopsy, 58–61
　　skin scrapings, 57–58
　differential diagnosis, 16t
　etiology and pathogenesis, 3–8
　　alterations in microflora in, 6–7
　　anatomy of skin and, 3, 5i
　　cutaneous pathogens, 6
　　normal microflora of skin and hair, 3–6
　　zoonotic potential, 7
　future developments, 89–91
　　evaluation for immunocompetency, 89
　　general considerations, 89
　　manipulation of microbial flora, 89–90
　　modification of host response, 90
　　new antibacterial products, 90
　German shepherd dog, 16t, 52–53
　management of
　　assessment of, 73
　　coexisting problems complicating, 76t
　　factors complicating, 75–76
　　general considerations, 63
　　immunomodulatory therapy, 71–73
　　initial, 73
　　overview of, 63–74
　　recurrent, 83–87, 83t
　　systemic antibiotic therapy, 63–69
　　topical antibacterial therapy, 69–71
　overview, 1–2
　　frequency of occurrence, 1
　　predilections, 1–2
　pressure-point, 51–52
　recurrent, 77–82
　　management of, 83–87
　superficial, 27–39
　　bacterial folliculitis, 30–35, 31i
　　impetigo, 27–30, 28i
　　spreading pyoderma, 35–39, 36i
　surface pyoderma, 21–26
　　intertrigo, 22–25
　　mucocutaneous pyoderma, 25–26
　　pyotraumatic dermatitis, 21–22
　susceptibility and host response, 9–13
Pyotraumatic dermatitis, 16t, 20, 21–22, 80, 80t
Pyotraumatic folliculitis, 16t, 20, 47–49

R

Recurrent canine pyoderma, 77–87
　deep, 81–82
　general causes, 77–80, 79t
　　bacterial hypersensitivity, 79
　　immunodeficiency, 79–80
　　nonstaphylococcal pyoderma, 80
　　persistent underlying skin disease, 78–79, 78t
　　resistant strains of S. intermedius, 80
　general considerations, 77
　idiopathic, 82
　management of, 83–87
　　extended regimens of antibiotic therapy, 85–87, 86t
　　immunomodulatory therapy, 84–85
　　topical antibacterial therapy, 84
　　underlying diseases and other contributing factors, 83–84
　superficial, 81, 81t
　surface, 80–81, 80t
Rifampin, 66, 68–69

S

Sarcoptic acariasis
   and recurrent canine pyoderma, 78, 78t
Sebaceous adenitis
   and recurrent canine pyoderma, 78t, 79
Secondary skin lesions
   general clinical findings, 19–20
Shampoos, antibacterial
   for canine pyoderma, 69–71, 84
Skin biopsy
   in canine pyoderma, 58–61
Skin, canine
   anatomy of, 3, 5i
   normal microflora of, 3–6
Skin-fold pyoderma, 16t, 20, 22–25
Skin scrapings
   in canine pyoderma, 57–58
Soaks, antibacterial, 70–71
Spreading pyoderma, superficial, 35–39, 36i
Squamous cell carcinoma, solar-induced
   and recurrent canine pyoderma, 78t, 79
Staphage Lysate, 85
Staphylococcus intermedius
   as canine cutaneous pathogen, 6
   resistant strains of and recurrent pyoderma, 79t, 80
Sulfadimethoxine
   ormetoprim-potentiated, 67–68
Sulfonamides
   nonpotentiated, 65, 66
   potentiated, *see Ormetoprim and Trimethoprim*
Superficial bacterial folliculitis, 16t, 20, 30–35, 31i, 81, 81t
Superficial pyoderma, 27–39
   bacterial folliculitis, 30–35, 31i
   classification, 15t, 17
   differential diagnosis, 16t
   impetigo, 27–30, 28i
   recurrent, 81, 81t
   spreading pyoderma, 35–39, 36i
Superficial spreading pyoderma, 16t, 35–39, 36i, 81, 81t
Surface pyoderma, 21–26
   classification, 15–16, 15t
   differential diagnosis, 16t
   intertrigo, 22–25
   mucocutaneous pyoderma, 25–26
   pyotraumatic dermatitis, 21–22
   recurrent, 80–81, 80t
Susceptibility, to canine pyoderma, 9–13
   factors leading to, 9t
Systemic antibiotic therapy
   for canine pyoderma, 63–69
      basic principles, 63t
      clinical trials, 66
      culture and sensitivity studies, 65–66
      rational antibiotic selection, 66–69
      useful oral antibiotics, 64t, 67t

T

Tail-fold intertrigo, 16t, 22–25
Tetracycline, 65–66
Therapy, *see Management*
Topical antibacterial therapy
   for canine pyoderma, 69–71
      gels, creams, and ointments, 71
      shampoos, 69–70
      soaks and whirlpools, 70–71
   for recurrent canine pyoderma, 84
Treatment, *see Management*
Triclosan, 70, 84
Trimethoprim-potentiated sulfonamides, 64t, 65–68, 67t
   sulfadiazine, 68
   sulfamethoxazole, 68

V

Vulvar-fold intertrigo, 16t, 22–25

W

Whirlpools, antibacterial, 70–71

Z

Zoonosis
   potential of canine skin pathogens for, 7

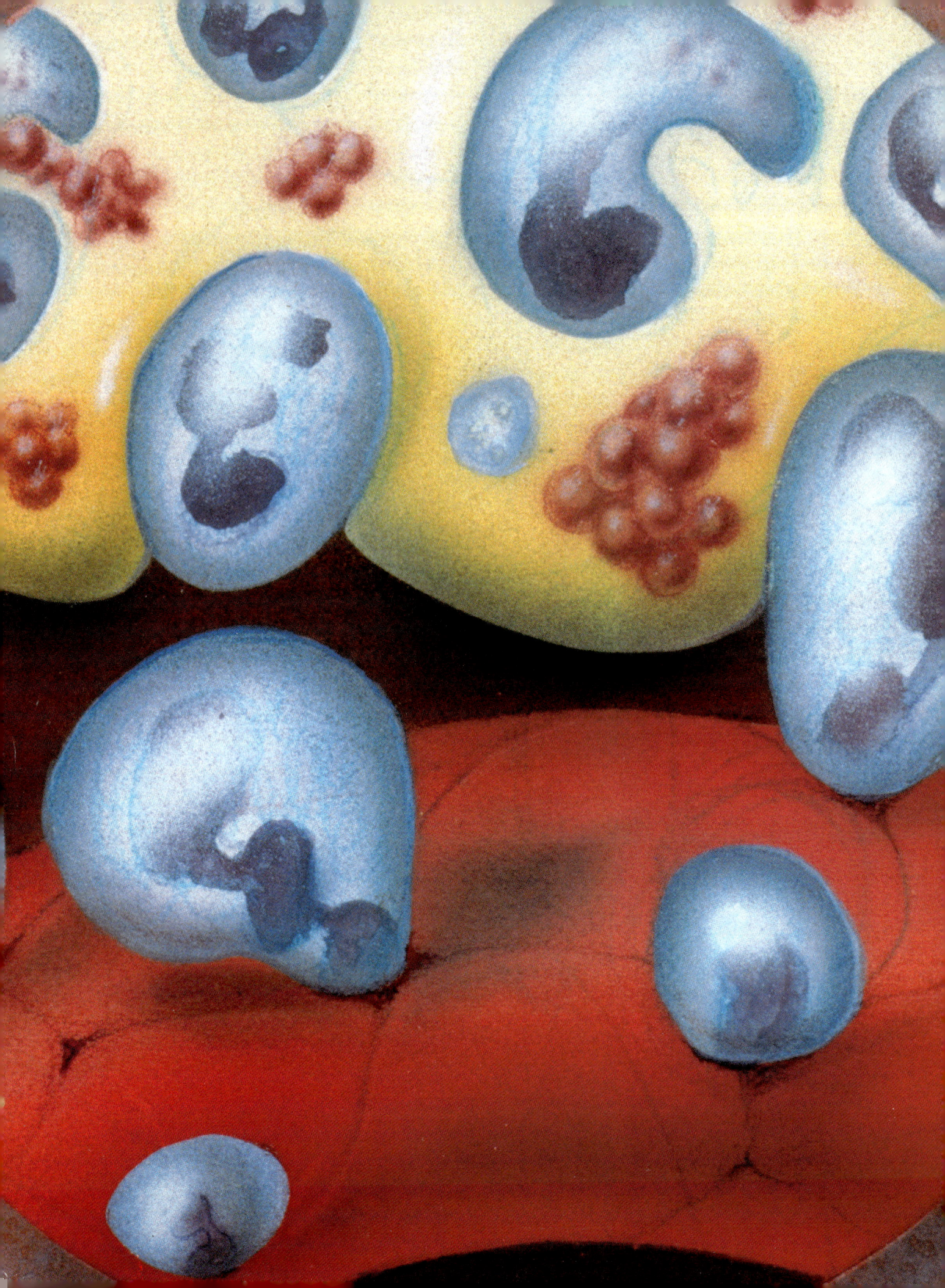